Stolen Memories

A Journey Through Alzheimer's

Maria L. Ellis, MBA

DEDICATION

To Claire,
whose strength, grace, and spirit continue to inspire us all.

To the caregivers,
who give so much of themselves in the face
of unimaginable challenges, embodying
love in its purest form.

And to the millions of individuals and families
navigating the journey of Alzheimer's,
may this book be a beacon of understanding,
hope, and compassion.

This is for you!

ADVANCE PRAISE

"A deeply moving and insightful book that captures the emotional, mental, and physical toll of Alzheimer's on families and caregivers. Maria L. Ellis offers not only understanding but also hope, practical guidance, and heartfelt wisdom."

— Dr. Namasivayam Gunatheesan, Malaysia

"Maria L. Ellis masterfully weaves together the personal and the universal, bringing much-needed awareness to the emotional complexities of Alzheimer's. This book is as informative as it is profoundly touching."

— Antonio Segna, Italy

"Raw, honest, and beautifully written, *Stolen Memories* serves as both a tribute to those battling Alzheimer's and a lifeline for caregivers searching for answers, support, and solace."

— Wei La Femina, Florida

"For anyone facing the long, painful goodbye that Alzheimer's brings, this book is an invaluable resource. It offers not only knowledge but also the emotional support caregivers so desperately need."

— Dr. Rosanna De La Cruz, Holistic Endocrinologist, New York

"A deeply personal yet universally relatable book that provides solace, understanding, and practical tools for families struggling with Alzheimer's. Ellis' words are a gift to caregivers everywhere."

— Dr. Catalina Matiz, California

TABLE OF CONTENTS

Foreword i

Preface 1

Chapter 1: The Thief of Memories: Understanding Alzheimer's Disease 3

Chapter 2: A Heartbreaking Disconnect: The Family's Struggle with Recognition Loss 7

Chapter 3: Lost Identity: The Disorientation of Alzheimer's for the Affected Person 13

Chapter 4: The Hidden Costs: Emotional, Mental and Financial Toll on Families 23

Chapter 5: A Global Perspective: How Different Cultures Approach Alzheimer's Disease 33

Chapter 6: The Fragility of Lucid Moments: Why Alzheimer's Patients Can't Care for Themselves 43

Chapter 7: Building Your Care Team and Caring for the Caregivers. 53

Chapter 8: Navigating the Alzheimer's Journey – Key Milestones and Medical Recommendations 61

Chapter 9: Taking Action – Advocacy Steps to Challenge Stigma 67

Chapter 10: Leveraging Technology for Alzheimer's Care 75

Chapter 11: Legal and Ethical Challenges: Navigating Alzheimer's Decisions 81

Chapter 12: The Future of Alzheimer's: Hope in Medical Discoveries 91

Chapter 13: Beyond One-Size-Fits-All: The Rise of Personalized Alzheimer's Therapies 99

Chapter 14: What Are the Ethical Considerations of Using AI and Technology in Alzheimer's Care?   105

Chapter 15: How Are Emerging Therapies, Like Gene Editing or Stem Cell Treatments, Being Explored for Alzheimer's Care?   131

Acknowledgments   153

About the Author   155

Thank You!   157

FOREWORD

Alzheimer's disease is an unrelenting adversary, robbing individuals of their memories, identities, and connections to the world around them. It is a cruel condition that not only reshapes the lives of those diagnosed but also profoundly affects their families and caregivers. The emotional and mental toll of watching a loved one slip away, piece by piece, is an experience that is as painful as it is universal.

In *Stolen Memories: A Journey Through Alzheimer's*, Maria L. Ellis, BBA, MBA, shares a deeply personal yet widely resonant story of navigating the challenges of this devastating disease. With honesty, compassion, and insight, she chronicles the heartbreaking moments of recognition loss, the struggles of caregiving, and the unbreakable love that persists even as memories fade. Her words reflect not only the pain of this journey but also the resilience, strength, and hope that can be found in the midst of suffering.

As a healthcare professional committed to understanding and improving brain health, I have both experienced and witnessed firsthand the impact that Alzheimer's has on individuals plus their families. While science continues to search for cures and more effective treatments, stories like Maria's serve as essential reminders that those living with Alzheimer's are still here, still deserving of love, dignity, and support.

Through my years of clinical practice, I have witnessed an increasing number of patients suffering from brain-based disorders, including Alzheimer's, dementia, and cognitive decline. The frustration of patients and their families is palpable, as traditional medicine often falls short in providing real solutions.

As a student of neuroscience during the 1990s, nicknamed the 'decade of the brain' and now as a practicing physician anesthesiologist who routinely, intentionally interrupts neural pathways, I have remained committed to advancing my knowledge, attending seminars, and staying at the forefront of brain-based wellness. However, beyond the science, what truly matters is the human connection—the ability to offer comfort, guidance, and hope to those struggling with conditions like Alzheimer's.

This book is more than a memoir—it is a companion for those who are facing the daily realities of Alzheimer's, offering comfort, validation, and guidance. Whether you are a caregiver, a family member, or someone seeking to understand the profound effects of this disease, *Stolen Memories* will touch your heart and inspire you to cherish every moment with the ones you love.

Maria's heartfelt words remind us all of the importance of compassion, advocacy, and the unwavering commitment to preserving the dignity of those affected by Alzheimer's. May this book bring solace and strength to all who embark on this journey.

Dr. Cathleen Peterson-Layne, PhD, MD
Founder, BEing inCredible
Retired Professor of Anesthesiology

PREFACE

As I lay me down to sleep...

A memory as vivid as those words themselves.

Our mother Claire, a young woman of just thirty, had her hands full raising six children - a blended family of five boys and one girl. Yet, no matter how long the day or how exhausted she must have felt, she never failed to kneel beside our beds each night, guiding us in prayer.

"If I should die before I wake..."

These words remain etched in our hearts, untouched by time. Those whispered words, the warmth of our mother's presence, the gentle cadence of her voice - these are the fragments of love that Alzheimer's will never steal from us. **"I pray my Lord, my soul to take."**

Alzheimer's is a cruel thief, robbing its victims of their identity and their families of the person they once knew. It doesn't just take memories, it takes recognition, connection, and shared history, leaving behind a painful void. We have witnessed this firsthand, watching our mother journey through the twilight of her life, slipping further into a world where the past and present blur, and where familiar faces become strangers.

This book is not just about the science of Alzheimer's. It is about love, the loss, and the resilience required to navigate this devastating disease. It is a story of grief, yes - but also of gratitude. Because while Alzheimer's may take away names, places, and timelines, it can never erase the love that binds us.

To everyone walking this path with a loved one, we see you! I understand your sorrow, your exhaustion, and you're longing to hold onto the person(s) slipping away before your eyes. This book is for you!

And to our mother - thank you. For the prayers, the love, and the memories that even time cannot take.

With much love and appreciation,

Your Children,
Steve, Tom, and Joan

CHAPTER 1:
THE THIEF OF MEMORIES:
UNDERSTANDING ALZHEIMER'S DISEASE

"Alzheimer's is a cruel thief, slowly stealing the essence of a person. But the heart remembers what the mind forgets."

-- Unknown

Alzheimer's disease is more than just a medical condition - it's a complex and devastating reality that affects millions of individuals and their families. In this chapter, I want to help you understand what Alzheimer's truly is, from the neurological changes that lead to memory loss to the genetic, environmental, and lifestyle factors that contribute to its development. By exploring the science behind the disease, we can begin to make sense of the heartbreaking symptoms we see in our loved ones and approach their care with greater knowledge, empathy, and support.

For me, this understanding is deeply personal. Claire, my husband's mother, is now ninety-four years old. For over ten years, we've watched her slowly slip away from the vibrant person she once was. Her journey through Alzheimer's has been painful to witness, but it has also driven me to share this knowledge with others - so that families like ours and yours can better comprehend what's happening inside the brain of someone with this disease. The more we know, the more compassionate and effective we can be in helping those we love.

Why Does Alzheimer's Happen? The Causes of This Disease

Even though we understand how Alzheimer's progresses in the brain, the question of why it happens is more complex. Alzheimer's is influenced by a mix of genetic, environmental, and lifestyle factors, and while Claire's situation is unique, many families share similar experiences.

- **Genetics**: For some people, including those with early-onset Alzheimer's, genetics play a significant role. However, in cases like Claire's, which appeared later in life, genetic factors still matter, but they work alongside other influences. People with a variant of the APOE gene - specifically APOE ε4 - are at a higher risk of developing the disease. If Claire carries this gene, it could explain part of her risk, but it's not the full story.

- **Environmental and Lifestyle Factors**: Claire's long life has been shaped by many factors including her health, her activity level, and even the stress she's faced over the years. Conditions like high blood pressure, diabetes, and heart disease can increase the risk of Alzheimer's because what's good for the heart is often good for the brain. Conversely, a lifestyle filled with physical activity, mental stimulation, and strong social connections can help protect against cognitive decline. Claire's experiences, good or bad, likely contributed to where she is today.

How Alzheimer's Affects More Than Memory

We tend to think of Alzheimer's as a disease of memory loss, but its effects reach far beyond that. Claire's changes may seem primarily focused on her ability to remember, but as her brain functions deteriorate, other skills and senses are also affected. This can make Alzheimer's especiallyfrustrating for families, who often wish their loved one could still engage with them in the same ways.

Language and Communication Problems

You've probably noticed that Claire struggles to find words or follow conversations. This isn't just memory loss - it's a breakdown in the brain's ability to process and retrieve information. She might recognize what she wants to say but can't express it in words, which can lead to frustration for both her and those around her.

Impaired Reasoning and Judgment

As Alzheimer's continues to impact Claire's brain, tasks that once seemed simple - like making decisions about what to wear or whether to eat - become overwhelming. You might see her struggling to make basic choices or becoming confused about everyday things. This happens because the frontal lobe, responsible for judgment and planning, is also affected by the disease.

Personality Changes

Alzheimer's can cause someone's personality to shift dramatically. If Claire has become more anxious, withdrawn, or even angry at times, it's because the disease is changing the way she perceives the world. These personality changes are not a reflection of who she was, but rather how Alzheimer's is altering her brain's ability to regulate emotions.

A Hopeful Future: The Search for a Cure

While we can't reverse Claire's condition, we're living in a time when more is being done to understand and combat Alzheimer's than ever before. Medications like donepezil and memantine can slow down some symptoms for a time, but researchers are constantly working on new treatments. Some of the most promising developments include drugs that target amyloid plaques and tau tangles directly, and research into how lifestyle changes and early interventions can reduce the risk of Alzheimer's altogether.

Alzheimer's is a thief that takes memories, identity, and independence, leaving loved ones struggling to hold on to fleeting moments of connection. Understanding what happens in the brain can help us navigate this journey with greater compassion and patience. Though we can't stop what's happening to Claire, we can continue to support her with love, respect, and as much dignity as possible, knowing that the moments we share - no matter how brief - are still meaningful.

CHAPTER 2:
A HEARTBREAKING DISCONNECT:
THE FAMILY'S STRUGGLE WITH
RECOGNITION LOSS

Alzheimer's disease is often referred to as the "long goodbye," and nowhere is this more profoundly felt than in the erosion of recognition - the cornerstone of human connection. In this chapter, I will share our personal journey with Claire, my ninety-four-year-old mother-in-law and my husband Stephen's beloved mother. Claire has been living with Alzheimer's for over a decade. Once the vibrant matriarch of our family, she now exists in a world where familiar faces often become strangers.

Claire's kindness and warmth have always defined aspects of her character. Over the years, we've shared countless pleasant dinners, weaving memories from laughter and lively conversations. We often reminisce with her about old friends, cherished family gatherings, funny mishaps, her favorite recipes, and beloved travel destinations. For fleeting moments, we see glimpses of the Claire we knew - her face lighting up as she recalls a story or laughs at a shared joke. Yet, these moments are bittersweet, as they are often punctuated by confusion and disorientation.

One evening stands out in my mind, a poignant illustration of the heartbreaking disconnects. We were seated around the dinner table, sharing stories from our day, when Claire turned to Stephen and asked, "And who are you again?" The room fell silent. Stephen's expression froze for a moment before he gently responded, "It's me, Mother. Stephen."

Her brow furrowed as she searched his face, and then she shook her head slightly, as if trying to clear a fog. "Are you my son?" she said hesitantly. My husband replied, "Guilty as charged, Mother. I am your son, Stephen..." and then they both smiled.

That evening, the weight of Alzheimer's pressed down on all of us. The sorrow in Stephen's eyes was unmistakable, a mix of pain and resignation. For a son, being unrecognized by the woman who gave him life is at once a unique and profound heartbreak. For me, as an observer and a daughter-in-law, that moment underscored the disease's devastating reach - how it doesn't just steal memories but also the bonds that define us.

The Ripple Effect on Family

The emotional toll of Claire's recognition loss extends beyond Stephen. Her grandchildren, once greeted with joyous hugs and beaming smiles, now face moments where she looks at them as strangers. They try to engage her with stories of school and their hobbies, but her responses are often distant or unrelated, as if she's grasping at threads of a nonexistent tapestry.

Her son Stephen and his sister Joan take turns every two weeks taking care of Claire, assisted by three different caregivers: Joyce, Lillian, and Deborah. Each of them is such a blessing. They help take care of Claire under the supervision of Stephen and Joan. Often, Claire is in her own world based on prompting from her children, and increasingly less often, she recalls a few humorous stories from their childhood.

Claire was a school psychologist in Warren County, Ohio. She was raised in Franklin and was married three times, giving birth to three children: Stephen, Joan, and Thomas. All of Claire's children have shown her immense love and care throughout her Alzheimer's journey, remaining compassionate despite her loss of identity and stolen memories.

Despite the challenges, there are moments of unexpected beauty. One afternoon, while flipping through an old photo album, Claire pointed to a picture of herself as a young woman and said, "I think she looks happy. Do you know her?"

I replied, "That's you, Claire. You look beautiful."

She smiled faintly and said, "I hope I was nice." It was a fleeting moment of self-awareness, tinged with sadness and vulnerability. Yet, it was also a reminder of her enduring spirit and the essence of who she is - kind, thoughtful, and deeply human.

This is my goal for you - to help you find those moments, no matter how fleeting, so you can support your loved one with grace through this enduring process. While Alzheimer's can feel overwhelming, small, meaningful gestures can make a difference. We'll start with something simple, yet powerful - weekly rituals - that can bring both you and your loved one a sense of connection and peace.

Weekly Rituals

Maintaining dignity through weekly rituals is essential for both the person with Alzheimer's and their caregivers. These rituals offer familiarity and comfort, reinforcing identity and emotional well-being. However, as the disease progresses, adapting to these routines becomes increasingly necessary.

Identifying and Preserving Meaningful Routines

To preserve meaningful routines, caregivers can:

1. **Observe Preferences:** Take note of which activities bring joy or comfort, such as listening to a favorite song, engaging in gentle exercises, or participating in spiritual practices. Claire finds joy in listening to songs from Johnny Cash and Dolly Parton, and she especially enjoys listening to Bible hymns such as "That Old Rugged Cross,"

"Blessed Assurance," "I Surrender All," and "It Is Well with My Soul."

2. **Simplify Tasks:** Modify activities to align with the person's abilities, such as replacing intricate cooking tasks with simple food preparation or turning full-length books into short storytelling sessions.

3. **Use Sensory Cues:** Incorporate music, scents, or textures to maintain engagement, like playing familiar tunes during a morning routine or using aromatherapy to signal bedtime.

4. **Encourage Participation:** Allow the person to contribute to the ritual in a way that suits their capacity with minimal guidance. During Christmas time, my husband Stephen and I would decorate our Christmas tree, and we encouraged Claire's participation. She would let us know that she liked our Christmas decorations very much. Watching us decorate the Christmas tree brought her much joy.

Adapting Cherished Habits

As Alzheimer's advances, cherished habits may become challenging. Here are strategies for adjusting these routines while preserving their essence:

Mealtime Rituals

If using utensils becomes difficult, introduce easy-to-hold adaptive cutlery or switch to finger foods while maintaining favorite flavors.

Grooming and Self-Care

When independent grooming is no longer possible, guide their hand for brushing hair or washing hands, fostering a sense of participation. Every Friday, Claire has her hair done. Many times, Claire doesn't have the energy to get up from her couch, so her son Stephen tells her that they're going for ice cream. Somehow, the promise of a sweet treat gives Claire the motivation to walk to the car, aided by her son Stephen, her daughter Joan, or one of her caregivers.

Social Engagements

If large gatherings become overwhelming, arrange smaller, quieter visits with close family members to maintain a sense of connection. Every two weeks, Claire has her nails done, always opting for a French style. Nothing but the best for Mother. These small rituals provide her with a sense of normalcy and dignity, and they remind us of her enduring love for the comfortable habits of her past life.

Creative Outlets

If detailed artwork or knitting is no longer feasible, transition to simple finger painting or textured fabric swatches for tactile stimulation.

By proactively modifying these routines, caregivers can preserve the dignity and individuality of their loved ones, creating a sense of stability despite the uncertainties of Alzheimer's.

Coping with the Emotional Strain

Watching a loved one slip away in such a profound way is a grueling test of resilience. As a family, we've found solace in small rituals: playing her favorite music, cooking her cherished recipes, and surrounding her with familiar objects. These routines anchor her - and us - to a sense of continuity, even as the disease erodes her ability to connect.

We've also learned to find joy in the present, however fragmented it may be. Whether it's a spontaneous laugh, a moment of clarity, or simply holding her hand, we cherish these instances as gifts. For more stories, refer to Chapter 7: "Coping with Emotional Strain," which focuses on caregiver burnout.

A Shared Journey

Alzheimer's doesn't just affect the individual; it reverberates through the entire family, reshaping relationships and straining emotional endurance.

Our journey with Claire has been one of heartbreak and resilience, a delicate balance of mourning what was lost while embracing what remains - and I know this is a journey you, too, may be experiencing with your loved one. As you move forward into the next chapter, remember that while the path may be filled with sorrow, it is also interwoven with moments of profound love and heartfelt connection - experiences that transcend even the boundaries of memory.

CHAPTER 3:
LOST IDENTITY: THE DISORIENTATION OF ALZHEIMER'S FOR THE AFFECTED PERSON

"It's a terrible thing to lose your sense of self,
to forget who you are and what you love.
But even in the fog, fragments of who we are remain."

-- Unknown

Alzheimer's disease not only takes away memories but also the sense of self that we all hold onto so dearly. It's an unraveling that occurs slowly, sometimes so subtly that it's hard to pinpoint when it truly begins. For the person experiencing it, the world becomes unfamiliar, even hostile at times. Imagine waking up each day feeling as though everything and everyone around you is somehow wrong or out of place, but you can't quite explain why. This is the disorienting experience of Alzheimer's, where one's identity - so tightly bound to memories, relationships, and familiar routines - begins to fade, piece by piece.

The Loss of Self

At the core of Alzheimer's is the gradual loss of one's sense of identity. Identity is shaped by our memories, our connections to the people we love, and the routines and experiences that form our daily lives. As Alzheimer's progresses, it strips away these building blocks of who we are.

For someone like Claire, my husband's mother, who has lived with Alzheimer's for over ten years, the changes have been profound. Early in the disease, Claire could still remember details about her childhood and share stories from decades ago. But gradually, even those long-held memories began to fade. She would mistake her son for her husband or confuse her current home with one she lived in many years ago. Over time, these disconnects from reality made it harder for her to grasp who she was in the present moment.

There is an unsettling fear of losing the ability to recognize yourself in the mirror or remember the roles you've played in life - mother, friend, spouse. Imagine the anxiety of not being able to explain how you feel because the words are no longer within reach. For Claire and others like her, this is a constant source of fear and confusion. As memories vanish, so too does the ability to hold onto an identity that once felt secure and permanent.

While Alzheimer's is a disease of steady decline, it is punctuated by moments of clarity - fleeting glimpses when the fog lifts, and for just a second, the person seems to come back. These moments can be as heartbreaking as they are precious. Claire has had these moments, where for a brief time, she remembers something or someone clearly. In these moments, she might smile at a familiar face or speak a coherent sentence about the past. But just as quickly, those connections dissolve, leaving her more confused than before.

For the person with Alzheimer's, these brief periods of clarity can bring both relief and terror. They offer a painful awareness of what has been lost. Claire has often appeared startled after such moments, as if she suddenly realizes how much of her world has slipped away. It's in these moments that her fear is most visible, her eyes darting, searching for a connection to something familiar that is no longer there.

As the disease progresses, the world becomes increasingly foreign to someone with Alzheimer's. Familiar places feel alien, and people they've known for years seem like strangers. This disorientation extends to the most basic aspects of life - knowing what day it is, where they are, or even the purpose of daily activities like eating or dressing.

For Claire, simple tasks that were once second nature became confusing puzzles. She would sit at the dinner table, holding a fork, unsure of what it was for or how to use it. She would sit on her comfortable sofa, waiting for someone to take her "home," even though she had lived in the same house for years. Each day brought new confusion and, with it, new anxiety.

Imagine the exhaustion that must come from constantly feeling lost. This is what Alzheimer's does: it makes even the most familiar environments seem strange. It erodes the anchors that ground us in time and place, leaving the person adrift in a sea of uncertainty.

The Emotional Toll

The emotional impact of losing one's sense of self cannot be understated. Anxiety, frustration, and even anger are common reactions for those living with Alzheimer's. Claire would often be impatient with those around her - not from anger, but because her world had become incomprehensible. She couldn't understand why she was being asked to eat, bathe, or go to bed, and her confusion manifested itself as impatience. It's as though she was trying to assert control over a life that was slipping out of her grasp.

At other times, Claire would fall into long bouts of silence, as if retreating from a world that no longer felt safe. This emotional withdrawal is common among Alzheimer's patients. As they lose their ability to interact with the world in the way they once did, it becomes easier to retreat inward, to a place where there are fewer expectations and less confusion.

Fragments of Who They Were

Yet even as Alzheimer's takes away so much, pieces of the person still remain. Claire may not always recognize her family members, but sometimes a familiar scent or the sound of a favorite song can bring a fleeting smile to her face. These small moments remind us that, beneath the layers of confusion and fear, there are still remnants of the person we knew.

These fragments of the past - old memories, favorite activities, or cherished routines - can still bring comfort. They are like little beacons in the fog, brief connections to a time when things made sense. For Claire, we've found that listening to music from her younger years often helps soothe her anxiety. While she may not remember why the music is familiar, it seems to resonate somewhere deep within her, providing a small measure of peace. Religious hymns are often tied to Claire's formative experiences - such as attending church, family gatherings, or moments of spiritual reflection. These hymns are usually learned early and repeated frequently, which makes them more resistant to the memory loss caused by Alzheimer's. Even if Claire forgets many aspects of her life, the hymns she sang or heard regularly remain familiar and accessible.

Hymns like "The Old Rugged Cross" often carry profound emotional and spiritual meaning. They represent faith, hope, and comfort, which can evoke a sense of peace even in someone struggling with confusion. Claire, for example, might not remember why the song makes her feel safe, but the emotions it stirs remain intact. The melody and lyrics are associated with feelings of love, community, and a connection to her faith, which offer reassurance in moments of anxiety. Hymns that particularly resonate with Claire include "Amazing Grace," "How Great Thou Art," "In the Garden," and "What a Friend We Have in Jesus." These hymns connect with Claire in a way that little else can, offering a moment of familiarity and peace amid the confusion and fear that Alzheimer's brings. They help her find a connection to her past, her faith, and her sense of self, even when so much else has been lost.

As Alzheimer's progresses, the ways we help our loved ones need to change too. Here's where I offer some advice for how to best care for Claire - and yourselves as caregivers. Alzheimer's brings unpredictability, but creating a consistent daily routine can offer Claire comfort. Familiarity helps reduce confusion. If she knows what to expect each day, like when meals are served or what activities are planned, she's likely to feel less anxious. Communicating with Claire might require extra patience. Use short, simple sentences, give her time to process, and avoid correcting her if she says something wrong. It's less important to focus on the details of what she's saying and more on keeping the interaction calm and positive. As hard as it is, try to focus on the small joys of the present. Claire might not remember something that happened five minutes ago, but if she smiles at a photo, enjoys a song, or has a moment of clarity, cherish that. Alzheimer's is a disease that forces you to live in the moment with the person you love.

As we explore the journey through Alzheimer's disease in this book, each chapter provides a unique perspective on the disease, highlighting its complexity, the emotional and physical toll it takes on both patients and families, and the hope that exists through research and medical advancements.

Chapter 1 is the foundational chapter. We dive into the underlying causes of Alzheimer's, explaining the biological mechanisms such as the buildup of amyloid plaques and tau tangles that contribute to the disease. The chapter also addresses the genetic, environmental, and lifestyle factors that can increase the risk of Alzheimer's, providing a comprehensive overview of what leads to the gradual loss of memory and cognitive function. This chapter sets the stage by giving readers a clear understanding of the science behind the disease.

In Chapter 2, I write about how Alzheimer's doesn't just

affect the person diagnosed - it deeply impacts the entire family. In this chapter, we explore the emotional challenges families face, from coping with the grief of seeing a loved one lose their memories to the day-to-day stresses of caregiving. The emotional toll often includes feelings of frustration, helplessness, and guilt, and this chapter offers insight into how families can navigate these difficult emotions while providing support to their loved ones.

In Chapter 3, for the person living with Alzheimer's, the disease is a terrifying journey of losing one's sense of self. This chapter focuses on the confusion, fear, and frustration that accompany memory loss and cognitive decline. It examines how Alzheimer's erodes a person's identity, causing them to forget familiar faces, places, and even their own life story. The chapter also includes personal stories and anecdotes to illustrate the profound psychological impact the disease has on the individual.

In Chapter 4, I will write about how Alzheimer's imposes hidden financial and mental burdens on families. This chapter highlights the overwhelming costs of care, including long-term care facilities, in-home caregiving, and medical expenses. It also addresses the mental exhaustion that caregivers experience, emphasizing the need for shared caregiving responsibilities and external support. Through real-life examples, the chapter shows the significant sacrifices families make to care for their loved ones with Alzheimer's.

In Chapter 5, we explore how different cultures view and handle Alzheimer's, including the role of family, the societal respect for elders, and how healthcare systems in various countries are responding to the growing challenge of dementia. By examining these diverse approaches, we can learn valuable lessons in Alzheimer's care and discover innovative solutions to improve the quality of life for those affected.

In Chapter 6, I share with you how Alzheimer's disease robs individuals of their ability to think clearly, make decisions, and remember even the most basic aspects of daily life. Even in the moments of apparent clarity - those precious, fleeting periods where a person with Alzheimer's seems to recognize loved ones or recall a piece of long-forgotten information - they remain unable to fully take care of themselves. This chapter delves into the reasons behind this, exploring the neurological, emotional, and practical barriers that prevent people with Alzheimer's from being self-sufficient, even when they experience lucid moments.

In Chapter 7, I write that caring for someone with Alzheimer's disease is an act of love, but it also comes with an immense emotional and physical toll. For the caregivers, whether they are family members or professionals, the responsibility of managing day-to-day challenges often leads to burnout, stress, and emotional exhaustion. Alzheimer's is a disease that doesn't just affect the person diagnosed with it; it changes the lives of those who care for them as well.

In Chapter 8, we explore the essential recommendations that the medical profession offers to families coping with a loved one's Alzheimer's diagnosis. This chapter will highlight the advice of doctors, specialists, and caregivers on how to navigate the emotional, physical, and logistical challenges of caring for someone with Alzheimer's. The focus will be on practical strategies for providing the best care while maintaining the family's well-being. This chapter will also emphasize the importance of support networks, communication with healthcare professionals, and understanding when and how to seek additional care options, such as assisted living or hospice care.

In Chapter 9, I write about how Alzheimer's disease touches the lives of millions of people across the globe, yet for many years it remained misunderstood, shrouded in stigma, and often talked about in hushed tones. As more people and families come forward with their stories, and as public figures raise their voices, awareness of Alzheimer's has grown, leading to important shifts in how the disease is perceived by society. This chapter examines how increased visibility and education combat Alzheimer's stigma, showcasing pioneering efforts.

In Chapter 10, I continue to seek answers in the battle against Alzheimer's disease. Technology and artificial intelligence (AI) have emerged as transformative tools, reshaping how we approach diagnosis, care, and treatment. From monitoring cognitive decline in real time to developing sophisticated predictive models, advancements in technology are offering new hope for earlier detection and better care for those affected by the disease.

In Chapter 11, I write about how Alzheimer's disease not only affects the cognitive abilities of those diagnosed but also places a heavy burden on their families and caregivers to make important legal and ethical decisions. As the disease progresses and individuals lose the ability to express their wishes or make informed choices, caregivers must take on the responsibility of ensuring their loved one's rights, dignity, and well-being are maintained. These decisions often touch upon sensitive issues, such as medical treatment, guardianship, financial control, and end-of-life care.

In Chapter 12, I write about how Alzheimer's is often described as a slow, relentless thief - a disease that steals memories, independence, and a sense of self. For families like Claire's, who have spent over a decade witnessing their loved one fade away, the darkness of Alzheimer's can feel overwhelming. Yet amid this darkness shines real hope - emerging from research laboratories and dedicated scientists. In this chapter, we explore the current medical advancements that are shedding light on the path forward, offering hope to those affected by Alzheimer's and their families.

In Chapter 13, I share ideas about where the future of Alzheimer's treatment may lie - in the promise of personalized medicine. By tailoring therapies to the unique genetic, environmental, and lifestyle factors that influence each individual's experience with Alzheimer's, researchers hope to develop more effective treatments that can slow the progression of the disease or even prevent it.

In Chapter 14, I write that by adopting a more multifaceted approach - targeting not only amyloid but also tau, inflammation, and other pathways - researchers can develop more effective treatments. Improved diagnostic tools, early intervention, diverse clinical trials, and collaborative research networks will be critical for accelerating breakthroughs. With these insights, the Alzheimer's research community is better equipped to overcome the challenges of the past and bring us closer to finding a cure for this devastating disease.

Conclusion

This book will offer a comprehensive journey through the many facets of Alzheimer's disease, from the scientific understanding of the condition to the personal, emotional, and practical challenges it presents. Each chapter builds on the previous one, providing a holistic view of Alzheimer's, along with stories of resilience, hope, and the advancements being made toward better treatments and care. Ultimately, this book is not only a resource for understanding Alzheimer's but also a guide for families and caregivers to navigate the difficult path ahead with knowledge, compassion, and hope for the future.

So, let's get to work.

CHAPTER 4:
THE HIDDEN COSTS: EMOTIONAL, MENTAL AND FINANCIAL TOLL ON FAMILIES

*"You will face many defeats in life but
never let yourself be defeated."*

-- Maya Angelou

Caring for a loved one with Alzheimer's disease is not only emotionally taxing; it can be a journey that drains families in many unexpected ways. The hidden costs of Alzheimer's often come as waves, each one taking a little more from caregivers and families: their time, energy, mental well-being, and financial stability. This chapter aims to shed light on the multi-layered burdens families face when caring for someone with Alzheimer's, highlighting the sacrifices made, the emotional toll, and the often-overlooked financial strain that compounds over time.

The Emotional Weight of Caregiving

At first, families often embrace the role of caregiver with love and determination. They want to do everything they can to help their loved one - after all, they've always been there for you. But as the disease progresses, the emotional weight of caregiving becomes heavier. For someone like Claire, who has lived with Alzheimer's for over a decade, the early stages brought frustration and confusion, but as the disease deepened, the emotional toll on her family intensified.

Watching someone you love slowly lose their memories, their ability to speak, and their independence creates a sense of grief that stretches over years. Unlike the sudden loss of a loved one, Alzheimer's is a slow goodbye, where every day brings a new challenge and another piece of the person slipping away. We have had to adjust to the reality that the woman we once knew no longer recognizes us. Though she is still physically present, the essence of who she was has faded. This ongoing emotional burden - known as ambiguous loss - can leave families feeling stuck between hope and despair.

The Importance of Shared Caregiving

Fortunately, Claire's family has been able to share the burden of caregiving. Claire's daughter has stepped in to help her brother, providing much-needed respite from the exhausting daily responsibilities. This shared caregiving arrangement has given her brother a chance to rest and recharge, allowing him to maintain his well-being while continuing to care for their mother.

Sharing the caregiving responsibilities has also helped prevent burnout. Alzheimer's caregiving can be an isolating and overwhelming experience, but by dividing the responsibilities, both siblings have been able to take time for themselves, which is critical in preventing emotional exhaustion. Their teamwork serves as a reminder that caregiving is not meant to be faced alone, and having a support system - whether family members, friends, or professional caregivers - makes an enormous difference.

The Mental Exhaustion of Caregiving

Even with shared responsibilities, the mental exhaustion of caregiving is ever-present. The constant vigilance required to care for someone with advanced Alzheimer's - helping them dress, eat, bathe, and stay safe - leaves little room for rest or mental recuperation. Caregivers often find themselves feeling isolated and overwhelmed as the demands of caregiving become all-consuming.

We have experienced sleepless nights, checking on Claire to ensure she hasn't wandered or become disoriented. These restless nights take their toll, leaving caregivers feeling drained, anxious, and often overwhelmed. Over time, this constant state of stress can lead to **caregiver burnout**, a state of physical, emotional, and mental exhaustion that can make it difficult to continue providing care.

The mental health effects extend beyond exhaustion. Caregivers of Alzheimer's patients are more likely to experience depression, anxiety, and chronic stress. It's not uncommon for caregivers to neglect their health, prioritizing their loved one's needs above their own. The strain of trying to be constantly present and emotionally available while coping with the sadness of watching someone decline can lead to feelings of guilt, resentment, and helplessness.

The following are some practical strategies and real-world examples that make the journey of caregiving more relatable and manageable.

Caregiving can feel like it takes over every aspect of life, especially with a progressive disease like Alzheimer's. Many caregivers struggle with maintaining their sense of self as the demands of caregiving grow. However, it is crucial for caregivers to preserve their identity beyond their role as a caregiver.

Setting Boundaries

One of the most effective strategies is setting boundaries and giving yourself permission to prioritize self-care. This doesn't mean neglecting your loved one - it means recognizing that you, too, have needs. Caregivers can maintain a sense of identity by scheduling time for themselves, whether it's engaging in hobbies, socializing with friends, or pursuing personal goals. Carving out time for exercise, meditation, or even reading can provide a much-needed mental break and help caregivers reconnect with who they are outside of caregiving.

Accepting Support

Another important aspect is asking for help. Accepting support, whether through respite care, family assistance, or community programs, allows caregivers the space to breathe. Claire's family, for example, shared the caregiving load, ensuring her son had time to recharge and focus on his own life, thus preventing burnout.

Caregivers can also benefit from joining support groups, where they can share their experiences and frustrations with others who understand. These groups provide a vital space to voice personal concerns, seek advice, and gain emotional support. Connecting with other caregivers reminds individuals that they are not alone and reinforces the importance of maintaining a life outside of caregiving.

Mixed Emotions

After years of devotion, the loss of a loved one with Alzheimer's can bring up a complex mix of emotions. Many caregivers experience profound grief, as they've lost not only the physical presence of their loved one but also the person they used to know. This grief can be complicated by the fact that, in some ways, caregivers have been grieving throughout the disease's progression as they watched their loved one fade away bit by bit - what is known as anticipatory grief.

At the same time, some caregivers may feel a sense of relief - a feeling that is often accompanied by guilt. The intensity of Alzheimer's caregiving can be overwhelming, and when the journey ends, it's natural to feel a release from the relentless responsibilities and emotional toll. These conflicting emotions are normal, and caregivers should allow themselves the space to feel both grief and relief without judgment.

Long-term emotional effects can also include a loss of purpose. After years of dedicating themselves to caregiving, some individuals struggle with finding a new routine or sense of identity. Post-caregiver support groups orcounseling can be beneficial during this transition, helping families process their grief while rediscovering what brings them joy and fulfillment beyond caregiving.

Guilt and resentment are common emotions in caregiving, particularly when the demands of caring for someone with Alzheimer's start to overwhelm the caregiver. Many caregivers feel guilty for not doing enough, for getting frustrated, or for needing time away. Others may feel resentment toward the endless tasks and the ways caregiving has taken over their lives.

One way to manage these feelings is to acknowledge and accept them without self-judgment. Caregiving is hard, and feeling negative emotions doesn't make someone a bad caregiver - it makes them human. Expressing these feelings through journaling or talking to a trusted friend or therapist can help caregivers process their emotions instead of letting them build up.

Realistic Expectations

Another strategy is setting realistic expectations. Caregivers often feel guilty when they can't "fix" the situation, but Alzheimer's is a disease that cannot be reversed. Instead of aiming for perfection, caregivers should focus on doing their best each day, understanding that they are giving their loved one the care and support they need in this difficult time.

Self-compassion is equally important. Just as caregivers show compassion to their loved ones, they must extend that same kindness to themselves. Recognizing that it's okay to need breaks, to make mistakes, and to feel overwhelmed allows caregivers to maintain their compassion for their loved one without being consumed by guilt or resentment.

Practical Strategies for Shared Caregiving

Expand the shared caregiving section with actionable strategies:

Create a Schedule: Use shared calendars like Google

Calendar or apps like CareZone to coordinate shifts and appointments.

Divide Responsibilities: Assign tasks based on strengths (e.g., one family member handles finances while another provides day-to-day care).

Leverage Technology: Use video monitoring systems, medication reminder apps, or online grocery delivery to streamline caregiving efforts.

Hold Regular Family Meetings: Reassess needs, address challenges, and redistribute tasks as necessary.

Managing the Costs: Support and Resources

Despite these challenges, families don't have to face them alone. There are resources available to help manage the emotional, mental, and financial burdens of Alzheimer's care:

Support Groups

Caregivers benefit greatly from connecting with others who are going through similar experiences. Support groups, both in-person and online, offer a space to share stories, advice, and encouragement. Knowing that others are facing the same emotional and mental struggles can provide a sense of community and reduce feelings of isolation.

Respite Care

Respite care services allow caregivers to take a break from their responsibilities while ensuring their loved one is safe and well cared for. Whether for a few hours, a day, or longer, respite care can offer much-needed relief from the constant demands of caregiving.

Financial Assistance

Depending on the country and region, financial aid may be available for Alzheimer's care. Government programs, grants, or non-profit organizations often provide support for caregiving costs, long-term care, or medical bills. It's important for families to research and explore all available options.

The Financial Burden of Alzheimer's Care

One of the most under-acknowledged aspects of Alzheimer's care is the financial strain it places on families. The costs of managing Alzheimer's often accumulate quietly until one day they become overwhelming. These costs go far beyond medical bills and include:

Long-Term Care Facilities

As Alzheimer's progresses, many families reach a point where they can no longer provide the level of care needed at home. Placing a loved one in a memory care facility can provide the professional care they need, but the costs are steep - often thousands of dollars per month. For Claire's family, the decision to place her in a facility may loom in the future, but for now, they continue to provide care at home, sharing the responsibilities of managing the emotional and financial strain.

In-Home Care

Families who wish to keep their loved ones at home often hire professional caregivers to help with daily tasks. These services, while invaluable, can cost hundreds of dollars per week, adding up quickly. Claire's family has already had to explore this option to provide some relief during especially challenging periods.

Lost Income

Many caregivers, like Claire's son and daughter, reduce their working hours or even leave their jobs altogether to care for their loved one. This lost income adds to financial strain, especially when combined with the rising costs of care.

Medical Bills and Medications

Alzheimer's patients often require various medications to manage symptoms like anxiety, depression, or agitation. While insurance may cover some, out-of-pocket expenses add up over time, especially when specialized treatments or therapies are involved.

Home Modifications

Families often need to make adjustments to their homes to ensure the safety of their loved one with Alzheimer's. Installing safety rails, locks, or alarms to prevent wandering, along with other necessary changes, comes with additional costs.

The financial burden is a silent weight that can leave families feeling financially depleted and emotionally worn out. This is why many caregivers describe Alzheimer's as not only a personal and emotional challenge but also a significant financial one.

Caring for a loved one with Alzheimer's can be emotionally overwhelming, but the financial burden can also be significant. However, you don't have to navigate this journey alone - there are financial assistance programs that can help ease the strain.

Government Assistance Programs

Several federal and state programs provide financial support for individuals with Alzheimer's and their caregivers. Programs like **Medicare, Medicaid, Supplemental Security Income (SSI), and veteran benefits** can help cover medical expenses, home care, and long-term care services.

Medicare covers hospital stays, doctor visits, and limited home health care but does not typically cover long-term nursing home care. However, Medicare Advantage plans may offer additional benefits, such as adult day care services or caregiver support.

Medicaid provides long-term care coverage for those with limited financial resources, including nursing home care and in-home assistance. Each state has different eligibility requirements, so it's essential to check your local Medicaid program.

Supplemental Security Income (SSI) offers financial aid to elderly or disabled individuals with limited income and resources, helping to cover basic living expenses.

Veterans' Benefits through the Department of Veterans Affairs (VA) may offer additional financial support to veterans and their spouses, including Aid and Attendance benefits, which help cover the costs of in-home care, assisted living, or nursing home care.

Exploring these financial resources can make a significant difference in the quality of care your loved one receives. I encourage you to research these options, speak with a financial advisor, or contact local agencies to determine what assistance your family may qualify for. The more support you can secure, the more you can focus on what truly matters - cherishing the moments with your loved one.

Conclusion

The hidden costs of Alzheimer's are far-reaching and often take families by surprise. The emotional weight, mental exhaustion, and financial strain of caring for a loved one with Alzheimer's can leave families feeling depleted. Yet, even amid these challenges, there is resilience. Families find strength in love, in shared responsibilities, and in the knowledge that they provide care with compassion and dedication. Alzheimer's may defeat memory, but it doesn't have to defeat the spirit of the family.

As caregivers and loved ones, it's essential to acknowledge these burdens while also seeking support and resources to help lighten the load. Alzheimer's is a difficult journey, but it's one where no family has to walk alone.

CHAPTER 5:
A GLOBAL PERSPECTIVE: HOW DIFFERENT CULTURES APPROACH ALZHEIMER'S DISEASE

"We are more alike, my friends, than we are unalike."
-- Maya Angelou

Alzheimer's disease knows no boundaries; it affects individuals and families worldwide, crossing cultures, languages, and economic statuses. Yet the approaches to Alzheimer's care, family responsibility, and elder dignity vary dramatically across cultures, revealing both our shared humanity and distinctive social values. From deeply ingrained respect for elders in some cultures to advanced healthcare systems in others, each culture offers unique perspectives on how to handle Alzheimer's disease. Understanding these cultural differences can provide valuable insights into caregiving practices, support networks, and societal attitudes toward aging and memory loss.

In this chapter, we explore how different cultures view and handle Alzheimer's, including the role of family, the societal respect for elders, and how healthcare systems in various countries are responding to the growing challenge of dementia. By examining these diverse approaches, we can learn valuable lessons in Alzheimer's care and discover innovative solutions to improve the quality of life for those affected.

The Role of Family in Alzheimer's Care

The primary burden of Alzheimer's care falls to families in many cultures, revealing deep tensions between traditional values and modern healthcare systems. The way families embrace this role varies across the globe, influenced by cultural values, traditions, and societal expectations.

East Asia: Filial Piety and Family Duty

In East Asian cultures, such as China, Japan, and South Korea, the concept of filial piety - a deep-rooted respect for one's elders and the obligation to care for them - is central to how Alzheimer's care is approached. Traditionally, the elderly are cared for at home by their children or extended family members. This centuries-old expectation now collides with urbanization and modernization, creating painful choices for families navigating both filial responsibility and economic necessity.

In China, for example, multi-generational households are common, and it is expected that children will care for their aging parents. In fact, China passed a law in 2013 requiring adult children to visit their elderly parents regularly, reflecting the cultural importance of family caregiving. However, as China rapidly urbanizes and more young people move to cities for work, this tradition is being challenged, leading to a growing demand for professional care facilities.

Similarly, Japan, with one of the world's fastest-aging populations, also places a strong cultural emphasis on family caregiving. However, Japan has also innovated in Alzheimer's care, establishing a comprehensive long-term care insurance system that provides support for families caring for elderly relatives at home or in specialized facilities.

Southern Europe: Family Ties and Community Support

In Mediterranean countries like Italy, Greece, and Spain,

family bonds are incredibly strong, and caring for aging parents is considered both a privilege and a duty. Families in these cultures often take a more collective approach to caregiving, with multiple family members, including extended family, sharing the responsibility of caring for a loved one with Alzheimer's.

In Italy, for example, it is common for elderly individuals with dementia to live with their children or close relatives, and professional caregiving is often seen as a last resort. This approach is deeply tied to the values of familismo, which prioritizes family over individual needs. Despite this strong tradition of family caregiving, Mediterranean countries are beginning to face challenges similar to those in East Asia, as younger generations migrate to urban areas, leaving families caught between cultural expectations and demographic realities. Italy's response - innovative daycare centers and community support systems - represents a hybrid model that preserves family involvement while acknowledging new social patterns.

Societal Respect for Elders and Memory Loss

Cultural attitudes toward aging and memory loss play a significant role in how societies view Alzheimer's disease. In some cultures, memory loss and cognitive decline are viewed as a natural part of the aging process and are met with compassion and understanding. In others, Alzheimer's may carry more stigma, leading to isolation and reduced access to care.

Indigenous Communities: Memory Loss as Part of the Life Cycle

Indigenous communities worldwide often interpret memory loss through spiritual frameworks that honor rather than medicalize cognitive changes. Many Native American tribes, for example, continue to revere elders experiencing memory loss, viewing cognitive changes as transitions within life's sacred cycle rather than as pathologies requiring clinical intervention.

The Maori people of New Zealand similarly view aging as a time of life when spiritual connections deepen, and the loss of memory is sometimes seen as part of a journey to the afterlife. While these perspectives offer a compassionate view of aging, they can also present challenges when it comes to accessing modern healthcare for Alzheimer's treatment. Balancing traditional beliefs with modern medical care requires cultural sensitivity and respect for Indigenous worldviews.

Western Societies: Growing Awareness and Advocacy

In contrast, many Western societies, such as the United States, Canada, and the United Kingdom, have historically struggled with the stigma surrounding Alzheimer's and dementia. Memory loss was often misunderstood, and those with Alzheimer's were sometimes isolated from their communities or placed in long-term care facilities with limited engagement.

However, over the past few decades, public awareness of Alzheimer's has grown significantly, thanks in part to advocacy groups and public figures sharing their personal experiences with the disease. These societies are now shifting toward person-centered care models that prioritize the individual's dignity, autonomy, and remaining capabilities - representing a significant departure from institutional approaches that once defined Western eldercare. Support networks, memory care programs, and social activities are being developed to help individuals remain engaged in their communities for as long as possible.

Healthcare Approaches to Alzheimer's Care

While cultural values shape family involvement in Alzheimer's care, the healthcare systems in different countries also play a critical role in determining the level of support available for patients and caregivers. Some nations have developed comprehensive, state-supported systems, while others rely more heavily on private care.

The Scandinavian Model: Comprehensive Public Support

Scandinavian countries like Sweden, Norway, and Denmark are often cited as models for elderly care, including Alzheimer's care. These countries have extensive public healthcare systems that provide a range of services for individuals with Alzheimer's, including home care, daycare centers, and specialized dementia care facilities. The focus in these countries is on maintaining the highest possible quality of life for individuals with Alzheimer's, with the state taking on much of the financial burden.

In Sweden, for example, individuals with Alzheimer's are entitled to free or heavily subsidized healthcare, and municipalities are responsible for providing long-term care services. Families can access home care support, including nurses, personal assistants, and respite care, allowing individuals with Alzheimer's to stay in their homes for as long as possible.

The U.S. and Canada: Mixed Public and Private Models

In North America, Alzheimer's care is often a mix of public and private systems. In the United States, while Medicare provides some coverage for Alzheimer's care, many families find themselves paying out of pocket for long-term care, memory care facilities, or in-home caregivers. As a result, financial strain can be a significant challenge for American families dealing with Alzheimer's.

Canada, by contrast, has a publicly funded healthcare system, but the availability and quality of Alzheimer's care vary by province. While there are excellent memory care programs and resources in many areas, access to care can be limited in rural or remote regions. Canadian provinces are increasingly adopting age-friendly policies to improve care for seniors, including those with Alzheimer's, by creating more community-based resources and integrating dementia-friendly training for healthcare workers.

Innovations in Alzheimer's Care: The Dutch Dementia Villages

One of the most innovative approaches to Alzheimer's care comes from the Netherlands, where dementia villages have been developed to provide a unique living environment for individuals with Alzheimer's. The most famous example is Hogeweyk in the town of Weesp, where residents with dementia live in a specially designed village that resembles a traditional Dutch community. The residents live as independently as possible, with caregivers disguised as shopkeepers, neighbors, or friends. The village design deliberately reduces anxiety by eliminating confusing medical equipment, institutional uniforms, and clinical settings. Instead, familiar architectural elements, seasonal decorations, and everyday activities provide cognitive anchoring points that reduce agitation and medication dependence among residents. This adds crucial clinical reasoning behind the innovative approach.

This model focuses on maintaining a sense of normalcy and autonomy for individuals with Alzheimer's, allowing them to live in a secure environment while engaging in meaningful activities. The success of Hogeweyk has inspired similar projects around the world and highlights the importance of innovative thinking in Alzheimer's care.

What We Can Learn from Global Approaches

There is no one-size-fits-all solution to Alzheimer's care, but by examining the diverse approaches taken by different cultures and countries, we can identify key lessons:

Respect for Elders Is Universal

Whether in East Asia, Southern Europe, or Indigenous communities, respect for elders is a common theme across cultures. Ensuring that individuals with Alzheimer's are treated with dignity and compassion, regardless of their cognitive decline, should be a priority for every society.

The Importance of Family and Community

While some cultures place a stronger emphasis on family caregiving, others provide more institutional support. The best approaches blend family involvement with community-based resources and professional care, ensuring that caregivers are supported and that individuals with Alzheimer's receive the best possible care.

Innovation and Flexibility

Countries like the Netherlands are leading the way in innovative Alzheimer's care, but other countries can benefit from adopting flexible, person-centered care models that prioritize quality of life. Whether through dementia-friendly communities, technological solutions, or integrated healthcare systems, there is always room to improve how we care for those with Alzheimer's.

Caregiving approaches vary across cultures, and integrating these diverse perspectives can enhance the quality of care for Alzheimer's patients. Here are some cross-cultural caregiving practices that families can adopt:

East Asian Family Decision-Making Models

In many East Asian cultures, caregiving is a family-centered responsibility, often involving collective decision-making. Families can hold regular meetings to discuss care plans and assign roles, ensuring that responsibilities are shared rather than falling on a single caregiver. In Japan, the concept of oyakoko (filial piety) emphasizes caring for elders as a moral duty. Adopting this perspective can encourage younger family members to stay involved in caregiving tasks.

Mediterranean Multi-Generational Care Strategies

Mediterranean families, particularly in Italy and Greece, emphasize multi-generational living arrangements where elders remain integrated into daily life. If possible, they arrange living spaces that accommodate multi-generational interactions, such as shared meals or structured social time with younger family members. Italian families often involve elders in everyday activities, such as helping prepare meals or telling family stories. Encouraging these small roles fosters a sense of purpose and belonging.

Indigenous Holistic Care Approaches

Many Indigenous communities view elder care as a communal responsibility, incorporating spiritual and nature-based healing. They often include outdoor activities and natural surroundings into caregiving, such as spending time in a garden or engaging in culturally significant rituals. Some Native American tribes use storytelling as a way for elders to pass on wisdom. Encouraging Alzheimer's patients to share memories, even if fragmented, can provide emotional fulfillment.

Scandinavian Dementia-Friendly Communities

In Scandinavian countries, cities and neighborhoods are designed to support dementia patients, emphasizing autonomy and accessibility. They modify the home environment to be more dementia-friendly, such as using clear signage, maintaining a consistent layout, and reducing clutter to minimize confusion. Denmark has specialized dementia villages where residents can move freely within a safe, structured environment. While not always feasible, families can create similar structured spaces within the home.

By integrating these global caregiving strategies, families can create a more supportive and enriching environment for loved ones with Alzheimer's, ensuring they remain valued members of the family and community.

Conclusion

As Alzheimer's rates climb globally, we have a rare opportunity to transcend cultural boundaries and create caregiving models that incorporate the best elements from diverse traditions: the family cohesion of East Asia, the community integration of Mediterranean societies, the spiritual respect of Indigenous approaches, and the technological innovations of Western healthcare. The future of Alzheimer's care lies not in choosing between family or institutional support but in creating culturally responsive systems that honor both universal human dignity and distinct cultural values.

CHAPTER 6:
THE FRAGILITY OF LUCID MOMENTS: WHY ALZHEIMER'S PATIENTS CAN'T CARE FOR THEMSELVES

"Memory is not just the imprint of the past time upon us; it is the keeper of what is meaningful for our deepest hopes and fears."
-- Rollo May

Alzheimer's disease systematically dismantles a person's ability to think clearly, make sound decisions, and remember even the simplest routines of daily life. Even in the moments of apparent clarity - those precious, fleeting periods where a person with Alzheimer's seems to recognize loved ones or recall a piece of long-forgotten information - they remain unable to fully take care of themselves. This chapter delves into the reasons behind this, exploring the neurological, emotional, and practical barriers that prevent people with Alzheimer's from being self-sufficient, even when they experience lucid moments.

The Illusion of Lucidity

Lucid moments in Alzheimer's patients can be incredibly deceptive. For families, these moments often seem like glimmers of hope, as if their loved one has returned, if only for a short while. However, these moments are not indications that the person has regained their cognitive abilities or can resume normal functioning. Instead, they are brief lapses where the disease momentarily allows access to memories or connections that have otherwise been eroded.

During lucid episodes, an individual may recognize a familiar face, recall a specific event, or even ask questions that seem surprisingly coherent. However, these moments are generally short-lived and often leave the person disoriented or confused afterward, which can heighten their frustration. More importantly, while they might experience a fleeting sense of awareness, the underlying cognitive impairments remain. Basic tasks like remembering medications, understanding the time of day, or even identifying their surroundings remain beyond their grasp

Why Lucid Moments Don't Restore Independence

Even though a person with Alzheimer's may have brief periods of awareness, the brain damage caused by the disease prevents them from regaining the full mental capacity needed to care for themselves. Alzheimer's affects various parts of the brain responsible for different functions such as:

Memory Recall

Even during apparent clarity, the extensive damage to the hippocampus - our brain's memory command center - prevents reliable recall of recent events. A person might clearly remember their childhood home but have no recollection of eating lunch just thirty minutes earlier or whether they've taken vital medication.

Judgment and Decision-Making

Alzheimer's affects the frontal lobe, the part of the brain responsible for decision-making and planning. A person might feel clear-headed for a short time but will still lack the ability to make safe or appropriate choices about their health, finances, or safety. For example, they might forget the danger of leaving the stove on or wandering outside alone.

Physical Coordination and Safety

As Alzheimer's progresses, the brain's control over physical abilities also deteriorates. This means that even if someone can momentarily remember something or recognize someone, they may not be able to physically take care of themselves. Tasks like dressing, bathing, and managing personal hygiene require not only mental clarity but physical coordination, which Alzheimer's compromises.

Emotional Dysregulation

Alzheimer's often causes emotional swings, from depression to agitation, which further complicates self-care. During lucid moments, these emotions can resurface in overwhelming ways, making it hard for individuals to focus on anything other than their emotional distress.

Understanding Lucid Moments and Their Limitations

Lucid moments in Alzheimer's patients are brief periods where cognitive clarity and memory seem to return. These fleeting instances can provide emotional relief for caregivers and families, yet they also come with inherent limitations that must be acknowledged.

What Are Lucid Moments?

Lucid moments occur unpredictably, often triggered by familiar surroundings, music, or interactions with loved ones. During these episodes, individuals may a) recognize family members and recall past events; b) communicate more clearly than usual; and c) express emotions in ways not typically seen in their daily state. These complex dynamics are perfectly illustrated by an interaction between Claire and her granddaughter Taylor. During a hair appointment, Claire experienced a sudden moment of lucidity that revealed how her sense of self remained intact, even as her memory failed: "Taylor has a memorable story about a day at Taylor's nail salon with her grandma, Claire, whom she affectionately calls Nana. In the midst of her hair appointment, she suddenly became lucid and glanced down at her outfit, puzzled. 'What am I wearing?' she exclaimed. Taylor gently reminded her, 'Nana, you picked this out this morning and said you liked it.' Nana gave Taylor a surprised look and replied, 'Ugh, I would never!' Nana's reaction stemmed from the fact that her outfit wasn't what she typically wore. Claire was always the epitome of class, favoring black, cream, white, pearls, and elegant silk blouses paired with tailored trousers. However, on that day, she was dressed in a floral print that didn't quite suit her refined style."

The Emotional Impact on Caregivers

While these moments offer a glimpse of the person's former self, they can also create false hope. Caregivers should approach lucid moments with appreciation but manage expectations by understanding a) lucidity does not indicate cognitive recovery; b) these moments may be followed by deeper confusion; and c) over-reliance on such episodes can lead to emotional exhaustion.

Making the Most of Lucid Moments

To cherish these rare interactions, caregivers can:

Stay Present

Engage in conversation without questioning the validity of their statements. For example, Claire's daughter, Joan, watched her mother gradually slip away. The cherished moments they spent reminiscing, which once brought them closer, began to turn into a source of strain. Often confused, Claire started to ask about the whereabouts of her own deceased mother, Garnet. Joan learned through experience that honesty wasn't always the best approach. Now, Joan simply reassures her by saying that Garnet is at her house and that they'll see her later today!

Capture Memories and Create Familiar Environments

Playing favorite music, showing old photos, or using comforting scents can sometimes encourage lucidity.

Creating memorable sensory experiences can trigger moments of connection: Claire's ninetieth birthday celebration illustrates this perfectly. Though her memory was significantly compromised by then, the sensory spectacle of an Elvis Presley impersonator created a moment of pure joy and clarity when we celebrated Claire's ninetieth birthday. The entire family gathered for this special occasion, but there was one guest who made it truly unforgettable - an Elvis Presley impersonator! He serenaded Claire with "Happy Birthday" and performed some of her favorite songs. Claire was in absolute disbelief that "Elvis" had come to her ninetieth birthday party just for her. To top it off, he presented her with a beautiful red scarf as a birthday gift. It was a truly memorable birthday celebration for Claire and for the family.

Recognizing the Limitations

Despite their significance, lucid moments do not alter the progressive nature of Alzheimer's. Understanding their limitations helps caregivers maintain realistic expectations and provide compassionate, patient-centered care.

By embracing these moments while recognizing their fleeting nature, families can find comfort in small victories without becoming emotionally overwhelmed by the disease's challenges.

The Cycle of Confusion and Fear

Even during their most lucid moments, people with Alzheimer's exist in a fractured timeline where past, present, and future blur together unpredictably. They might recognize that something is wrong but lack the cognitive framework to understand their condition, creating a terrifying loop of awareness and confusion. While they may recognize that something is wrong, they often cannot grasp the full extent of their illness. This realization can cause feelings of helplessness, anxiety, and fear. A common consequence is that they may resist help or become frustrated, thinking they are still capable of tasks they can no longer manage.

For instance, someone may believe they are still in control of their finances or that they can drive a car, even though their ability to navigate basic decisions has significantly declined. This misperception of their abilities creates a dangerous situation, one that caregivers must constantly monitor to keep them safe.

The Importance of Consistent Care

Ultimately, even during moments of apparent clarity, individuals with Alzheimer's cannot be left to care for themselves. The unpredictability of lucidity, combined with the permanent cognitive decline caused by the disease, requires constant supervision and support. Families often struggle with this realization, especially during moments when their loved one seems temporarily "back to normal." But it is in these moments of confusion - where the person believes they are fine but are not - that the risks of injury, neglect, or danger are most present.

Why Alzheimer's Patients Lose the Ability to Care for Themselves

Alzheimer's affects critical areas of the brain responsible for memory, reasoning, and motor skills. As the disease progresses, it disrupts the connections needed to complete daily tasks. This decline manifests in several ways:

- **Memory Loss:** Patients forget the steps involved in routine activities, such as making a meal or taking medication.

- **Cognitive Impairment:** Judgments become impaired, making it unsafe for patients to handle tasks like driving, using appliances, or managing finances.

- **Physical Decline:** Over time, motor skills and coordination deteriorate, leading to difficulty with dressing, eating, and personal hygiene.

- **Emotional Dysregulation:** Patients may

experience anxiety, agitation, or confusion, further complicating their ability to function independently.

The following stories from other families illustrate how even apparent moments of competence can mask profound cognitive challenges, underscoring why constant supervision remains essential regardless of temporary lucidity.

Grace's Morning Ritual: A Routine Forgotten

Grace was a retired librarian who had always prided herself on her meticulous morning routine. Her daughter, Emma, noticed the changes gradually.

"Mom, did you have breakfast?" Emma asked one morning.

"Of course," Grace replied, but the untouched cereal box and empty fridge told a different story. Emma soon realized her mother had forgotten not just to eat but how to prepare even the simplest meal.

On rare occasions, Grace would have a moment of clarity, pouring herself a glass of orange juice or buttering toast. But these glimpses of lucidity were bittersweet. They reminded Emma of the person her mother used to be while underscoring how much she had lost.

Robert and the Stove: A Dangerous Combination

Robert, a former engineer, was known for his logical mind and problem-solving skills. But as Alzheimer's progressed, his family discovered how dangerous his once-sharp mind could be.

One afternoon, Robert decided to make tea. He placed the kettle on the stove, but as he waited, he forgot why he was in the kitchen. Hours later, the burning smell alerted his wife, Linda, to the forgotten kettle.

"I was just trying to boil water," Robert said, frustration evident in his voice. Linda realized that while he remembered the task, the sequence of steps was beyond him. This incident led to their decision to disconnect the stove for safety.

Clara's Dressing Dilemma: Lost in Familiarity

Clara loved fashion and had always dressed impeccably. But one day, her granddaughter found her struggling to put on a simple blouse.

"Why can't this fit?" Clara asked, holding the garment upside down.

The confusion was heartbreaking. Clara no longer recognized how to align her arms with the sleeves or differentiate the front from the back. These tasks, once second nature had become insurmountable puzzles, leaving her staring at the fabric in frustration. The simple act of getting dressed, once an unconscious routine, now required gentle guidance and patient reassurance. Each morning, as she struggled with buttons and folds, the disease's silent cruelty became more evident--stealing not just memories but the ability to navigate even the most familiar rituals of daily life.

Setting Practical Boundaries and Improving Communication

Understanding the limitations of lucid moments helps caregivers establish necessary boundaries. When family members misinterpret these moments as signs of recovery, they may inadvertently create dangerous situations or unrealistic expectations. The following strategies help navigate these complex dynamics:

1. Setting Boundaries

- **Define Your Limits**: Identify what you can realistically do and communicate this clearly to others.

- Say No When Needed: It's okay to refuse additional tasks that compromise your well-being.

- **Establish Time for Yourself:** Schedule regular breaks or "off-duty" hours to recharge.

2. Communication Strategies

- **Be Direct but Compassionate**: Use "I" statements to express your feelings without placing blame. For example, "I need help with scheduling appointments; it's becoming overwhelming."
- **Utilize Family Meetings**: Regularly discuss care plans and delegate tasks during family meetings to ensure everyone shares responsibilities.
- **Document Agreements**: Write down family care responsibilities to avoid misunderstandings or disputes.

3. Navigating Family Dynamics

- **Acknowledge Different Perspectives**: Understand that family members may have varying emotional reactions to the caregiving process.
- **Stay Solution-Focused**: Shift conversations from blame to actionable steps. For example, "How can we ensure Dad gets more social interaction?"
- **Seek Mediation if Necessary**: A third-party mediator or counselor can help resolve conflicts among family members.

A Compassionate Journey for Caregivers

Caring for someone with Alzheimer's is an act of profound love, but it can also take a heavy toll. By adopting a holistic approach to self-care, caregivers can find balance, resilience, and renewed purpose. With proper boundaries, effective communication, and a commitment to their well-being, caregivers can continue their journey with strength and compassion, honoring the person their loved one once was while navigating the challenges of who they are now.

This chapter offers not only understanding but also practical tools, reminding caregivers that they are not alone and that their well-being is as important as the care they provide.

Conclusion

While the moments of lucidity can feel like a brief reconnection with the person they once were, the sad reality is that these are not signs of recovery or self-sufficiency. Alzheimer's causes irreversible damage that strips individuals of the ability to care for themselves, regardless of these fleeting periods of clarity. For caregivers and loved ones, it's crucial to recognize this and provide ongoing, compassionate support, even when it feels as though a part of their loved one has returned temporarily.

CHAPTER 7:
BUILDING YOUR CARE TEAM AND CARING FOR THE CAREGIVERS

"You can't pour from an empty cup.
Take care of yourself first."

-- Unknown

Caring for a loved one with Alzheimer's is never meant to be a solo journey, though many caregivers mistakenly shoulder the burden alone. To provide effective care while preserving your own well-being, assembling a reliable care team isn't optional - it's essential to build a reliable and effective care team. This section outlines a systematic approach to creating a sustainable support network, ensuring that both the patient and caregivers receive the assistance they need.

Step 1: Identify Key Team Members

Start by assessing who in your circle can contribute to the caregiving process. Potential team members may include:

- **Family Members** - Spouses, children, siblings, and extended family who are willing to share responsibilities.
- **Friends and Neighbors** - Those who can offer companionship, transportation, or emotional support.

- **Medical Professionals** - Doctors, nurses, and therapists who provide medical care and guidance.
- **Professional Caregivers** - Home health aides, respite caregivers, and assisted living staff.
- **Community and Support Groups** - Local Alzheimer's organizations, faith-based groups, and online communities.

Step 2: Define Roles and Responsibilities

Once potential members have been identified, clearly define their roles to avoid confusion and ensure balanced caregiving. Consider the following:

- **Primary Caregiver** - Oversees daily care, schedules medical appointments, and ensures basic needs are met.
- **Medical Liaison** - Communicates with doctors, manages prescriptions, and stays informed about treatment plans.
- **Emotional Support Lead** - Provides encouragement, organizes social activities, and helps with mental well-being.
- **Financial Manager** - Handles bills, insurance, and financial planning related to care needs.
- **Backup Caregivers** - Available to step in when the primary caregiver needs a break.

Step 3: Establish Communication and Coordination

A successful care team operates efficiently when communication is clear and consistent. Implement these strategies:

- **Regular Check-ins** - Schedule weekly or biweekly calls to update everyone on the care recipient's status.
- **Use of Technology** - Utilize shared calendars, group chats, or caregiving apps to coordinate

schedules and tasks.

- **Emergency Plan** - Create a plan for handling urgent medical or behavioral situations, ensuring all team members are aware of their responsibilities.

Step 4: Delegate Effectively

To prevent burnout, tasks should be shared appropriately. Consider the strengths and availability of each team member:

- Assign medical duties to those comfortable with healthcare management.
- Ask a neighbor or friend to assist with errands or social visits.
- Encourage family members who live far away to provide financial or administrative support.
- Consider professional respite care to provide relief for primary caregivers.

Step 5: Adapt and Reassess Regularly

Care needs will evolve as Alzheimer's progresses. Schedule periodic reviews to:

- Evaluate the effectiveness of current support structures.
- Adjust roles as necessary to meet changing demands.
- Introduce new resources or professional help when required.

Building a care team is one of the most impactful steps you can take in managing the challenges of Alzheimer's caregiving. By assembling a reliable support system, defining clear responsibilities, and maintaining open communication, caregivers can provide quality care while also preserving their well-being.

In this chapter, we will also focus on the needs of caregivers, who often sacrifice their well-being to care for their loved ones. We'll explore the emotional strain that caregiving can bring, strategies to avoid burnout, the importance of self-care, and the support systems available to help caregivers maintain their health and well-being.

The Emotional Toll of Caregiving

Caring for someone with Alzheimer's is a full-time job that goes far beyond the physical tasks of feeding, dressing, and bathing. It is emotionally demanding, as caregivers witness their loved ones slip away, often losing the ability to recognize them or remember cherished moments. This gradual decline can feel like a form of grief that never ends, as the person you once knew fades slowly from view.

For our family, this emotional toll has been a constant companion for over a decade. We have faced moments of overwhelming sadness as we have watched Claire struggle to remember her own life. The confusion in her eyes, the frustration when words fail her, and the moments when she seems lost in a world of her own - it all weighs heavily on us. We love Claire deeply, and the emotional burden of watching her decline feels unbearable at times.

Caregivers often experience a range of emotions - grief, frustration, guilt, and even anger. These emotions are normal, but they can be difficult to process, especially when caregiving feels like an endless cycle of giving without receiving. The emotional exhaustion is compounded by the relentless nature of Alzheimer's, which requires constant vigilance and care.

The Physical Strain of Caregiving

In addition to the emotional toll, caregiving can also take a significant physical toll. Lifting, moving, and assisting someone with Alzheimer's, particularly in the later stages, can be physically demanding. Caregivers often neglect their physical health as they prioritize the needs of their loved ones, skipping meals, losing sleep, and foregoing exercise. Over time, this neglect can lead to physical ailments like back pain, fatigue, and weakened immune systems.

For Claire's son Stephen and daughter Joan, this physical

toll manifests in a body that never fully rests. Their sleep fractures nightly as they instinctively wake to check their mother's whereabouts, ensuring she hasn't wandered into danger during periods of nocturnal confusion. These years of interrupted sleep, combined with the physical demands of helping her bathe, dress, and move safely, have left them in a state of depletion that caffeine can't fix, and weekends can't repair.

Caregiver Burnout: When the Cup Runs Dry

One of the biggest risks caregivers face is burnout - a state of physical, emotional, and mental exhaustion that can occur when the demands of caregiving overwhelm an individual's capacity to cope. Caregiver burnout can manifest as irritability, depression, anxiety, and physical symptoms such as headaches, digestive issues, or a weakened immune system.

Caregivers may also begin to feel disconnected from their loved ones, resentful of the constant demands, or guilty for wanting a break. These feelings can lead to a sense of isolation, as many caregivers struggle to find the time or energy to reach out for support.

For Claire's son Stephen, the crushing weight of caregiving responsibilities could have been unbearable, but the division of duties with his sister has created crucial breathing room. This shared approach allows each sibling periods of respite - time to reconnect with friends, tend to their health needs, and momentarily step out of the caregiver role. Their deliberate system of mutual relief has protected their mental and physical resilience in ways that isolated caregivers rarely experience.

Strategies for Avoiding Caregiver Burnout

While caregiving for a loved one with Alzheimer's can be incredibly demanding, there are strategies and resources available to help caregivers avoid burnout and maintain their well-being. Here are some ways caregivers can protect their health:

Ask for Help

Recognize caregiving as a team sport. Abandon the dangerous myth that devoted caregiving means doing everything yourself. Effective care for someone with Alzheimer's requires multiple people with complementary skills and availability. Whether recruiting family members, friends, faith communities, or paid professionals, distributing responsibilities isn't admitting failure - it's ensuring sustainable, higher-quality care.

Take Regular Breaks

Scheduling regular breaks is essential for maintaining both physical and emotional health. Respite care services, which provide temporary relief for caregivers, allow them to step away for a while, knowing their loved one is in safe hands.

Join a Support Group

Connecting with others who are going through similar experiences can provide emotional support and practical advice. Support groups, either in-person or online, offer a sense of community where caregivers can share their struggles and receive encouragement.

Set Boundaries

It's important for caregivers to set boundaries and be clear about their limitations. Saying "no" when necessary and creating time for self-care are essential for avoiding burnout. Caregivers should not feel guilty for taking time to rest or pursue their needs.

Practice Self-Care

Caregivers often forget to care for themselves. Simple practices like getting enough sleep, eating healthy meals, exercising, and engaging in activities that bring joy are vital for mental and physical health. Self-care is not selfish; it's a necessary component of being an effective caregiver.

Use Professional Support Services

Hiring professional caregivers or using respite care

services can provide significant relief. Professional caregivers are trained to handle the physical and emotional challenges of Alzheimer's care, allowing family members to focus on their well-being without guilt.

Consider Therapy

Caregiving can trigger a wide range of emotions, and it's important to have a space to process these feelings. Therapy or counseling can offer a safe environment to work through grief, anger, or guilt while also providing coping strategies for managing stress.

Stories of Caregivers Coping with Burnout

Claire's family has learned the importance of balance in caregiving. By sharing the responsibilities between her son and daughter, they have both been able to take breaks, rest, and avoid burnout. In one instance, when her son was feeling particularly overwhelmed, Claire's daughter stepped in to provide full-time care for a week, allowing him to take time for himself. This act of support helped him recharge and return to caregiving with renewed energy and patience.

Another caregiver, Mary, whose husband was diagnosed with early-onset Alzheimer's, initially tried to do everything herself. She managed his medications, kept up with his doctor's appointments, and assisted with daily tasks. But over time, the stress took a toll on her own health. She developed chronic headaches and started losing sleep. Eventually, Mary realized she needed help. She reached out to a local support group, hired a part-time caregiver, and began scheduling weekly outings with friends to recharge emotionally. These changes allowed her to continue caring for her husband without losing herself in the process.

The Importance of Support Systems

No one should have to face caregiving alone. A strong support system is essential for maintaining the caregiver's health and well-being. Support can come from family members, friends, local community services, or even online networks. Having someone to talk to, lean on, or step in when things get too overwhelming makes all the difference.

Caregivers should also take advantage of professional resources such as respite care, adult day care centers, and counseling services. These support systems are designed to provide caregivers with the tools they need to navigate the challenges of Alzheimer's care without losing themselves in the process.

Conclusion

The Alzheimer's caregiving journey represents one of life's most profound paradoxes: an act of extraordinary love that can simultaneously destroy the caregiver through neglect of self. By rejecting martyrdom and embracing the balanced approach outlined in this chapter - building care teams, establishing boundaries, and practicing radical self-compassion - caregivers create the sustainability necessary for this marathon of compassion.

By asking for help, taking breaks, and prioritizing self-care, caregivers can avoid burnout and continue to offer the compassionate, patient care their loved ones need. Alzheimer's may be a disease that takes, but through the right support and strategies, caregivers can give their best without losing themselves along the way.

CHAPTER 8:
NAVIGATING THE ALZHEIMER'S JOURNEY - KEY MILESTONES AND MEDICAL RECOMMENDATIONS

*"To care for those who once cared for us
is one of the highest honors."*

-- Tia Walker

Alzheimer's disease progresses through distinct stages, each requiring different levels of medical care and support. Understanding these stages helps families prepare for the evolving needs of their loved ones and ensure they have the right medical guidance at every step.

Initial Diagnosis: Understanding the Condition

Key Considerations

Confirming the diagnosis through cognitive assessments, neurological exams, and imaging tests such as MRI or PET scans. Discussing the prognosis with a neurologist or geriatric specialist. Developing an initial care plan that includes lifestyle modifications, medication considerations, and legal preparations.

Medical Recommendations

Establish a relationship with a neurologist or memory care specialist. Start medications that may help slow cognitive decline (e.g., cholinesterase inhibitors like Donepezil or Rivastigmine). Begin cognitive therapies and lifestyle changes, including a heart-healthy diet and regular physical activity. Discuss advance directives and legal planning with an attorney.

Early Stages: Adjusting to Cognitive Changes

During early stages, once-occasional memory lapses transform into persistent patterns that disrupt daily functioning. Subtle personality shifts - perhaps increased anxiety, withdrawal from favorite activities, or uncharacteristic irritability - often emerge before significant cognitive decline becomes apparent. This crucial window requires families to balance independence with safety, preserving the person's dignity while establishing supportive routines.

Medical Recommendations

Continue prescribed medications and monitor their effectiveness. Schedule regular checkups to track cognitive changes. Introduce occupational therapy to help with memory and daily functioning. Encourage participation in early-stage Alzheimer's support groups. Address mood changes with non-medication strategies, such as social engagement and structured routines.

Middle Stages: Increasing Care Needs

Greater difficulty with daily tasks such as dressing, eating, and personal hygiene. Increased confusion, agitation, and potential wandering behaviors. Caregivers will require more hands-on assistance and support.

Medical Recommendations:

Reevaluate medication effectiveness and adjust as needed. Consider behavioral therapies or, if necessary, medications for anxiety, agitation, or sleep disturbances. Transform the home environment to prevent wandering while preserving dignity - this includes disguising exits with curtains or decorative screens, installing door alarms or electronic tracking systems, and creating safe walking paths within the home that satisfy the urge to move without leading to dangerous areas.

Late Stages: Full-Time Care and End-of-Life Planning

The late stage brings profound vulnerability as cognitive abilities deteriorate significantly. Verbal communication often becomes minimal or nonexistent, though emotional awareness typically remains intact. The person now depends entirely on others for survival, facing heightened risks of aspiration pneumonia, pressure sores, and systemic infections. This stage requires caregivers to shift focus from rehabilitation to comfort-centered care while beginning the emotional work of anticipatory grief.

Medical Recommendations

Prioritize comfort-focused care, including pain management and palliative care options. Work closely with hospice or specialized dementia care teams. Continue discussions on feeding options, advance directives, and personal wishes. Provide emotional support for both the patient and caregivers, including counseling and bereavement services.

By understanding these key milestones in the Alzheimer's journey, families can proactively plan for medical and caregiving needs. Each stage presents unique challenges, but with the right support and preparation, families can ensure compassionate and effective care for their loved ones.

In this chapter, we will also explore the essential recommendations that the medical profession offers to families coping with a loved one's Alzheimer's diagnosis. This chapter will highlight the advice of doctors, specialists, and caregivers on how to navigate the emotional, physical, and logistical challenges of caring for someone with Alzheimer's. The focus will be on practical strategies for providing the best care while maintaining the family's well-being. This chapter will also emphasize the importance of support networks, communication with healthcare professionals, and understanding when and how to seek additional care options, such as assisted living or hospice care.

What are the most important medical recommendations for families supporting a loved one with Alzheimer's, and how can these strategies help ease the burden while ensuring the patient receives compassionate, effective care? Here are some of the most important medical recommendations that healthcare professionals offer to families caring for a loved one with Alzheimer's disease, along with strategies that can help ease the burden while ensuring compassionate and effective care:

Education and Understanding the Disease

Physicians consistently emphasize that knowledge functions as medicine in Alzheimer's care. Understanding the neurological basis of symptoms - recognizing that behaviors stem from brain changes rather than choice or stubbornness - transforms caregiving from a frustrating battle into a more compassionate journey. Families equipped with stage-specific knowledge can anticipate needs rather than merely react to crises, allowing them to preserve their emotional resources for the marathon of care ahead.

Early Planning for Legal and Financial Matters

Healthcare providers advise families to address legal and financial planning as early as possible, including setting up powers of attorney, living wills, and exploring long-term care options. Early planning alleviates stress and ensures that the wishes of the patient are honored as the disease progresses, preventing future conflicts and uncertainty. Work with a legal professional specializing in elder law to create a comprehensive care plan, ensuring the family is prepared for both medical and financial decisions.

Prioritize the Patient's Emotional Well-Being

Medical professionals stress the importance of

maintaining a comforting, familiar environment for the person with Alzheimer's to reduce stress and confusion. Familiarity and routine provide a sense of security for individuals with Alzheimer's, helping to manage their anxiety and emotional distress. Create a stable daily routine, fill the environment with familiar objects, and maintain a calm and reassuring tone when communicating with the patient.

Utilizing Professional Support and Resources

Doctors recommend families seek out professional caregiving services, support groups, and respite care to lighten the caregiving load and avoid burnout. Alzheimer's caregiving is physically and emotionally taxing. Professional support allows families to take breaks while ensuring their loved one receives the best care. Find local Alzheimer's support groups, in-home caregiving services, and respite care options. Joining a support network can provide emotional relief and practical advice from those who have been through similar experiences.

Practice Effective Communication Techniques

The medical community advises using simple, clear communication strategies to interact with Alzheimer's patients, focusing on patience and positive reinforcement. People with Alzheimer's may struggle with language, comprehension, and memory, so clear communication can reduce frustration for both the patient and the caregiver. Use short sentences, speak slowly, maintain eye contact, and offer reassurance with a calm tone. Avoid correcting the patient unnecessarily, as this can lead to distress.

Take Care of the Caregivers' Health and Well-Being

Healthcare providers frequently remind caregivers to prioritize their health - both physically and emotionally - to avoid burning out. Caregivers are at risk of physical and emotional exhaustion, which can lead to health problems and negatively affect the quality of care they provide. Maintaining personal well-being is essential for long-term caregiving. Regularly take breaks, seek counseling or therapy if needed, and maintain a support system of family and friends to share responsibilities. Incorporate exercise, hobbies, and relaxation techniques to manage stress.

Consider Assisted Living and Hospice Care When Necessary

Medical professionals encourage families to recognize when full-time caregiving at home is no longer feasible and to explore assisted living or hospice care options. As Alzheimer's progresses, the needs of the patient may surpass what family members can provide, and professional care facilities can offer specialized, round-the-clock care. Have regular discussions with the patient's doctor about the progression of the disease and plan for potential transitions to assisted living or hospice care when appropriate, ensuring that the patient's quality of life is prioritized.

Stay Up to Date on New Treatments and Clinical Trials

Doctors encourage families to stay informed about the latest research, treatments, and clinical trials related to Alzheimer's disease. Advancements in Alzheimer's research may lead to new therapies that can slow the progression of the disease or improve the quality of life for the patient. Work closely with the patient's healthcare team to explore potential treatments or clinical trials that may be beneficial. Regularly check in with Alzheimer's research organizations or foundations for updates on new medical discoveries.

Conclusion

It is my wish for the reader that by following these medical recommendations, families can provide compassionate and effective care for their loved ones while also managing the emotional and physical demands of caregiving. The combination of education, planning, communication, and self-care helps ensure both the patient and the caregivers are supported throughout the journey with Alzheimer's.

CHAPTER 9:
TAKING ACTION - ADVOCACY STEPS TO CHALLENGE STIGMA

"Awareness is the greatest agent for change."
-- Eckhart Tolle

While awareness of Alzheimer's disease has grown, stigma and misinformation persist. Instead of reiterating themes from the introduction, I want to provide you with a structured guide containing practical advocacy steps that will help you challenge stigma in your community. By moving from individual actions to broader community involvement, I'll show you how your personal advocacy can create meaningful change - both for your loved one and for others facing similar challenges.

Step 1: Educate Yourself and Others

Stay informed about the latest research, treatments, and care strategies for Alzheimer's. Share reliable information with family and friends to dispel common myths and misconceptions. Encourage open conversations about the disease to normalize discussions and reduce fear-based stigma.

Step 2: Support Caregivers and Patients

Offer practical assistance, such as running errands or providing respite care for caregivers. Engage with people living with Alzheimer's by treating them with respect, patience, and empathy. Promote caregiver support groups or community programs that provide relief andencouragement.

Step 3: Speak Up and Share Stories

Use social media to share real-life experiences, educational resources, and positive advocacy messages. Write opinion pieces or blog posts highlighting the realities of Alzheimer's and the importance of stigma reduction. Participate in podcasts, webinars, or public speaking events to spread awareness.

Step 4: Get Involved in Community Outreach

Partner with local organizations to host educational events and workshops. Encourage schools and workplaces to include Alzheimer's awareness programs in their health initiatives. Advocate for dementia-friendly policies in businesses and public spaces to make environments more inclusive.

Step 5: Advocate for Policy Changes

Contact lawmakers to support increased funding for Alzheimer's research and caregiver assistance programs. Get involved in legislative efforts to improve healthcare policies and long-term care options. Join national or local advocacy groups working to shape better public policies.

Step 6: Foster Inclusive Environments

Encourage businesses and public services to adopt dementia-friendly training for staff. Work with faith communities and social groups to create inclusive activities for people with Alzheimer's. Help establish memory cafés or safe spaces where patients and caregivers can connect and find support.

By following these structured advocacy steps, readers can actively participate in breaking the stigma surrounding Alzheimer's. Advocacy starts with individual actions but has the potential to ripple out into community-wide and national change. Everyone has a role to play in fostering a more understanding and supportive society for those affected by Alzheimer's.

Alzheimer's disease carries a heavy burden not just for those who experience it, but also for the families who care for them. One of the most painful aspects of this journey is the stigma that often surrounds the disease - misunderstandings, judgments, and silence that can isolate families when they most need support. In this chapter, I want to share my personal story with Claire to illustrate how stigma impacts lives and offer you practical steps to challenge misconceptions in your community.

Personal Reflections: Finding Strength Through Advocacy

For Claire and our family, challenging the stigma became an act of love. By sharing her story, we transformed uncomfortable silence into meaningful conversations. One of my most moving moments was when a neighbor approached me after a community event to say, "I didn't know how to act around Claire, but now I understand. Thank you for helping me see her as more than her diagnosis."

Those words reminded me that reducing stigma is about connection - seeing the person behind the disease and giving others the tools to do the same.

The Power of Collective Action

Reducing the stigma of Alzheimer's requires collective effort. By educating ourselves, speaking openly, and advocating for change, we can create a more compassionate and supportive world for those living with the disease and their families. Claire's journey taught me that while Alzheimer's takes much, it cannot erase the power of human connection.

I hope this chapter inspires you to become part of this vital change. Together, we can transform misunderstanding into empathy in our communities.

Alzheimer's disease touches the lives of millions of people across the globe, yet for many years it remained misunderstood, shrouded in stigma, and often talked about in hushed tones. As more people and families come forward with their stories, and as public figures raise their voices, awareness of Alzheimer's has grown, leading to important shifts in how the disease is perceived by society. This chapter explores the role of awareness and education in reducing the stigma surrounding Alzheimer's and highlights the ongoing efforts to change the way we talk about, treat, and support those affected by this devastating disease.

The Power of Awareness and Education

Awareness and education play critical roles in changing how society views Alzheimer's. Historically, Alzheimer's and other forms of dementia were often met with misunderstanding or fear. People suffering from the disease were sometimes dismissed as being "senile," and families faced a lack of information and support. However, as awareness of the disease has increased, so has the compassion and empathy shown toward those living with it.

Alzheimer's advocacy groups, healthcare professionals, and families like ours have made it our mission to educate others about the realities of the disease. We have worked to shift the narrative from one of hopelessness to one of understanding and support. This educational effort not only helps reduce the fear and stigma surrounding Alzheimer's but also encourages earlier diagnosis and intervention, which can make a significant difference in the quality of life for those affected.

Education Promotes Early Diagnosis

I have witnessed how awareness about early signs leads to timelier diagnoses and better outcomes for families like ours. People who are better informed are more likely to recognize the symptoms of memory loss, confusion, and changes in behavior, prompting them to seek medical advice. Early diagnosis not only helps in managing the disease but also gives families time to plan for the future and access resources.

Dispelling Myths

Education is essential in dispelling common myths about Alzheimer's. Many people still believe that memory loss is simply a natural part of aging, rather than recognizing it as a potential sign of a neurodegenerative disease. Awareness campaigns help people understand that Alzheimer's is not just about forgetting - it's a complex condition that affects cognitive functions, emotions, and behavior.

Challenging Stigma

Stigma often surrounds Alzheimer's because of the fear and misunderstanding associated with cognitive decline. By educating the public, we can reduce the stigma that prevents individuals from seeking help, discussing their symptoms, or receiving the support they need. The more we understand about the disease, the more empathy we can offer to those affected.

Famous Figures and Public Advocacy

One of the most effective ways to raise awareness about Alzheimer's is through the stories of well-known public figures who have battled the disease. When celebrities or high-profile individuals share their personal experiences with Alzheimer's, it puts a human face on the disease and brings it into the public consciousness in a powerful way.

Glen Campbell

One of the most prominent examples is country music legend Glen Campbell, who bravely shared his Alzheimer's diagnosis with the world in 2011. Instead of retreating from the public eye, Campbell embarked on a farewell tour, documenting his journey with the disease in the acclaimed film *Glen Campbell: I'll Be Me*. His openness about his struggles helped millions of people see the reality of living with Alzheimer's and sparked conversations about the need for more research and support.

Terry Pratchett

British author Terry Pratchett, known for his *Discworld* novels, was diagnosed with early-onset Alzheimer's in 2007. He became a vocal advocate for Alzheimer's awareness, writing about his experiences with the disease and pushing for more funding for dementia research. His advocacy brought attention to the fact that Alzheimer's doesn't just affect the elderly - it can strike people in their prime.

Sandra Day O'Connor

Former U.S. Supreme Court Justice Sandra Day O'Connor revealed that she had been diagnosed with dementia, possibly Alzheimer's, in 2018. Her announcement was significant, as she had been a symbol of strength and resilience throughout her career. Her decision to step away from public life due to Alzheimer's raised awareness about the challenges faced by people in positions of leadership who are affected by cognitive decline.

These public figures have helped to normalize conversations about Alzheimer's, showing that the disease can happen to anyone and that it doesn't diminish a person's worth or legacy. Their stories have inspired advocacy movements, raising funds for research and encouraging families to seek help.

The Impact of Awareness on Policy and Research Funding

As awareness of Alzheimer's has grown, so has the demand for more funding and resources to fight the disease. Increased public understanding has driven policymakers to address Alzheimer's as a major public health issue, leading to significant changes in how governments and healthcare systems approach Alzheimer's research and care.

Increased Research Funding

Thanks to the advocacy of organizations like the Alzheimer's Association and public figures, governments around the world have begun to allocate more resources to

Alzheimer's research. In the United States, funding for Alzheimer's research at the National Institutes of Health (NIH) has increased dramatically in recent years. This funding supports vital research aimed at understanding the causes of the disease, improving diagnosis, and developing treatments.

National and Global Action Plans

Countries are also developing national action plans to address Alzheimer's and dementia. In 2011, the United States launched the National Plan to Address Alzheimer's Disease, with the goal of finding a cure or effective treatment by 2025. Other countries, including the UK, Canada, and Japan, have also implemented national strategies to combat Alzheimer's. These plans focus on improving care, raising public awareness, and investing in research.

Legislative Support

Increased awareness has led to legislative action that benefits those living with Alzheimer's and their families. In many countries, laws have been passed to protect the rights of people with Alzheimer's, ensuring they have access to quality care and support. In the U.S., the Alzheimer's Accountability Act was passed to ensure that the NIH submits an annual budget to Congress, outlining the resources needed to meet the national Alzheimer's goals.

Reducing Stigma and Supporting Families

Reducing the stigma associated with Alzheimer's can have a profound impact on the lives of those affected by the disease and their families. When we challenge the misconceptions surrounding Alzheimer's, we open the door to greater understanding, empathy, and support. Here are a few ways reducing stigma can help:

Encouraging Open Conversations

One of the most significant benefits of reducing stigma is that it encourages open conversations about Alzheimer's.

Families are more likely to discuss the disease, seek a diagnosis, and share their experiences when they know they won't be judged or misunderstood. Open dialogue also helps caregivers feel less isolated and more supported.

Fostering Empathy

When society understands that Alzheimer's is a disease, not a failure of character or aging, it fosters empathy for those living with it. Instead of viewing Alzheimer's patients as burdens or liabilities, we begin to see them as individuals who deserve compassion, dignity, and support. This shift in perception can improve the quality of care they receive and reduce feelings of shame or guilt among patients and families.

Building Stronger Support Networks

Reducing stigma also helps build stronger support networks for families affected by Alzheimer's. When communities are educated about the disease, they are more likely to offer help, whether through local services, volunteer opportunities, or emotional support. This creates a safety net for caregivers, ensuring they don't have to face the challenges of Alzheimer's alone.

Conclusion

Alzheimer's is a disease that has long been surrounded by fear, misunderstanding, and stigma, but thanks to the efforts of advocates, families, and public figures, awareness is growing. With each story shared and each conversation started, we chip away at the barriers that prevent people from seeking help, sharing their experiences, and receiving the care they need.

Awareness is the greatest agent for change, and as we continue to educate ourselves and others about Alzheimer's, we move closer to a world where the disease is not only understood but also met with compassion, support, and ultimately, a cure. The future holds promise, and by raising awareness today, we can build a better tomorrow for those living with Alzheimer's and their families.

CHAPTER 10:
LEVERAGING TECHNOLOGY
FOR ALZHEIMER'S CARE

"The science of today is the technology of tomorrow."
-- Edward Teller

Technology is actively transforming daily life for Alzheimer's patients and their caregivers, creating safety nets that were unimaginable just a decade ago. This establishes technology as current reality rather than future potential.

From smart home systems to wearable devices, these innovations provide real-time support, improve safety, and help families navigate the challenges of caregiving more effectively.

Smart Home Technology: Making Innovation Accessible

Smart home technologies are no longer futuristic luxuries; they are practical tools that can ease the burden on caregivers while ensuring patient safety. These affordable systems include voice-activated assistants like Amazon Alexa that provide medication reminders with Claire's daughter's recorded voice - a familiar sound that generates better response rates than electronic tones. This adds specificity about how the technology actually works in practice: a) Automated lighting and motion sensors that reduce fall risks by ensuring well-lit paths at night; b) Smart locks and security systems to prevent wandering and notify caregivers if a door is left open; and c) Remote monitoring cameras that allow family members to check in without being intrusive. These solutions provide peace of mind and help patients maintain a sense of independence in familiar environments.

Assistive Technologies Supporting Alzheimer's Patients

Beyond smart home automation, various assistive technologies are transforming Alzheimer's care today. Unlike speculative advancements, these tools are currently in use, making a meaningful difference in patients' lives.

- **GPS Tracking Devices**: Wearable GPS devices like AngelSense or SmartSole help locate loved ones who may wander and provide alerts to caregivers in real time.

- **Medication Management Systems**: Electronic pill dispensers such as MedMinder and Hero provide reminders and dispense medication at scheduled times to prevent missed doses.

- **Digital Memory Aids**: Apps like MindMate offer cognitive exercises, music therapy, and reminders to help with daily tasks and memory retention.

- **Personal Emergency Response Systems (PERS)**: Devices like Life Alert and MobileHelp enable individuals to call for assistance with the push of a button.

By embracing the right technologies, caregivers can enhance safety, improve communication, and promote a better quality of life for their loved ones. While technology cannot replace human care, it serves as a powerful tool to support families navigating the complexities of Alzheimer's disease.

As we continue to seek answers in the battle against Alzheimer's disease, technology and artificial intelligence (AI) have emerged as transformative tools, reshaping how we approach diagnosis, care, and treatment. From monitoring cognitive decline in real time to developing sophisticated predictive models, advancements in technology are offering new hope for earlier detection and better care for those affected by the disease.

In this chapter, we will explore how these technologies are revolutionizing Alzheimer's care, with a focus on AI, wearable devices, smart home systems, and other innovations that are making a significant impact. These advancements are not just changing the way we treat Alzheimer's but also how we understand the disease, providing insights that could lead to breakthroughs in prevention and ultimately, a cure.

AI in Early Diagnosis and Predictive Models

One of the most exciting areas of advancement in Alzheimer's care is the use of artificial intelligence (AI) for early diagnosis and prediction. AI has the ability to analyze vast amounts of data, detect patterns that may be invisible to the human eye, and make predictions about the onset and progression of Alzheimer's with remarkable accuracy.

AI for Brain Imaging Analysis

AI is now interpreting brain scans with greater accuracy than many specialists, detecting microscopic changes in brain structure up to six years before clinical symptoms appear - potentially transforming Alzheimer's from a crisis-response condition to a manageable chronic disease. AI algorithms can detect subtle alterations in brain structure and function, such as the accumulation of amyloid plaques and tau tangles, much earlier than traditional diagnostic methods. This capability allows for earlier intervention, giving patients and families more time to plan and begin treatments that can slow cognitive decline.

Predictive Models for Alzheimer's Risk

Researchers are developing AI-based predictive models that analyze a combination of genetic, lifestyle, and environmental data to determine an individual's risk of developing Alzheimer's. These models use machine learning to sift through data from clinical trials, genetic studies, and patient histories to identify the factors most strongly associated with the disease. For instance, AI can analyze the presence of genetic markers, such as the APOE ε4 allele, combined with lifestyle factors like diet and exercise, to predict the likelihood of developing Alzheimer's decades before symptoms appear.

Cognitive Assessment Tools

AI is also being used to create digital cognitive assessments, which help track changes in memory, attention, and problem-solving abilities over time. These assessments, administered via apps or online platforms, use AI to detect patterns in a person's cognitive performance and flag any signs of decline. This continuous monitoring allows for a more personalized approach to care and ensures that interventions can be tailored to the patient's specific needs.

AI in Alzheimer's Research and Drug Discovery

In addition to its role in diagnosis and care, AI is transforming Alzheimer's research by accelerating the drug discovery process. By analyzing massive datasets from clinical trials and genetic studies, AI is helping researchers identify new targets for potential treatments and predict which drugs will be most effective for different patient populations.

Accelerating Drug Discovery

The greatest barrier to personalized Alzheimer's treatment isn't technological limitation but the bewildering complexity of the disease itself - a condition that emerges from a perfect storm of genetic vulnerability, inflammatory responses, vascular health, lifetime exposures, and dozens of other interacting factors unique to each patient. AI is being used to analyze data from thousands of clinical trials and genetic studies to identify patterns and potential drug targets that might have been overlooked. By predicting which compounds are most likely to succeed, AI can help researchers narrow down the options and speed up the development process. This has the potential to bring new treatments to the market faster, providing patients with more options for managing the disease.

Personalized Medicine

AI is also paving the way for personalized medicine in Alzheimer's care. By analyzing a patient's genetic makeup, lifestyle factors, and medical history, AI can predict how they will respond to different treatments. This allows doctors to tailor therapies to the individual, maximizing the chances of success while minimizing side effects. Personalized medicine has the potential to revolutionize Alzheimer's care by ensuring that patients receive the treatments that are most effective for their specific condition.

The Future of Alzheimer's Care: Integrating Technology into Everyday Life

As these technologies continue to evolve, they will likely become more integrated into the daily lives of people living with Alzheimer's and their families. The ultimate goal is to create a future where technology enhances independence, improves care, and offers earlier and more accurate diagnoses, all while supporting caregivers in their challenging roles.

The most effective Alzheimer's care emerges where cutting-edge technology meets human touch - when devices enhance connections rather than replace them, expanding the caregiver's capacity for genuine presence. This provides a more nuanced perspective on technology's role.

Whether through AI-powered diagnostic tools, smart home systems, or personalized treatments, technology is playing a crucial role in changing the way we understand and manage this disease. While the road to a cure may still be long, the innovations being developed today are making life better for those affected by Alzheimer's, offering hope for a brighter, more connected future.

The world of Alzheimer's care and research is being transformed by technology and artificial intelligence. From predicting risk and monitoring cognitive decline to enhancing daily life through smart home systems and virtual reality, these advancements are offering new ways to manage and understand Alzheimer's disease. As we look to the future, the continued integration of technology into Alzheimer's care will not only improve the quality of life for patients and caregivers but also bring us closer to the ultimate goal: preventing and curing this devastating disease.

CHAPTER 11:
LEGAL AND ETHICAL
CHALLENGES: NAVIGATING
ALZHEIMER'S DECISIONS

*"Do what you feel in your heart to be right - for
you'll be criticized anyway."*

-- Eleanor Roosevelt

Alzheimer's disease forces families to navigate a maze of
legal and ethical challenges that intensify as technology
increasingly intersects with caregiving decisions. This better
establishes the high stakes of these decisions.

From AI-driven monitoring devices to advanced
diagnostic tools, these innovations hold great promise but
also raise significant ethical concerns. This chapter explores
an ethical framework for integrating technology into
Alzheimer's care, examining issues of privacy, consent, and
the psychological impacts on patients and caregivers.

The Promise and Peril of Technological Interventions in Alzheimer's Care

Technological innovations are transforming Alzheimer's
care, offering tools that enhance safety, improve diagnostic
accuracy, and provide caregivers with much-needed
support. However, these advancements also present
complex ethical dilemmas that require careful consideration.

An Ethical Framework for Technological Intervention

To navigate the ethical complexities of technology in Alzheimer's care, caregivers must weigh every innovation against three critical values: privacy protection, meaningful consent, and psychological well-being.

1. Privacy Concerns

Challenges

Many technologies, such as wearable trackers or in-home monitoring systems, collect sensitive personal data, including movement patterns, medical information, and even emotional responses.

Ethical Questions:

- How is this data stored, and who has access to it?

- Can patients meaningfully consent to data collection if their cognitive abilities are impaired?

Guidelines for Ethical Use

- Implement robust data encryption and anonymization protocols.

- Ensure caregivers and legal representatives are fully informed about the scope of data collection and its purpose.

- Limit data access to authorized parties directly involved in the patient's care.

2. Consent Issues

Challenges

In the early stages of Alzheimer's, patients may still be able to provide informed consent. However, as the disease progresses, decision-making falls to caregivers or legal proxies.

Ethical Questions:

- How can we preserve the patient's voice in

decisions even as their ability to express it diminishes?

- What safeguards are in place to prevent misuse of consent by caregivers or third parties?

Guidelines for Ethical Use:

- Obtain consent early in the disease trajectory while the patient can still make informed decisions.

- Regularly reassess consent with the involvement of caregivers and healthcare providers.

- Use advance directives to outline the patient's wishes for future technological interventions.

3. Psychological Impacts on Patients and Caregivers

Challenges

Technologies designed to enhance safety, such as video monitoring systems, can feel intrusive or stigmatizing to patients. Similarly, caregivers may experience increased anxiety from constant alerts or data overload.

Ethical Questions

- How do we balance safety with the patient's right to dignity and emotional well-being?

- Can technological interventions inadvertently increase caregiver stress?

Guidelines for Ethical Use

- Design technologies that prioritize patient comfort and dignity, such as discreet monitoring devices.

- Offer caregivers training and resources to manage technological tools effectively.

- Include options for personalization, allowing families to choose the level of monitoring they feel comfortable with.

Case Study: AI-Driven Monitoring Systems

A family installs an AI-powered system in their home to monitor their father, who is in the mid-stages of Alzheimer's. The system alerts caregivers if their father wanders at night or forgets to turn off the stove. While technology improves safety, it also raises questions:

- Does constant monitoring erode the father's sense of independence?

- How is the collected data protected from misuse?

- What happens if the alerts overwhelm the family or caregivers?

When families examine these questions through our ethical framework, they transform abstract principles into practical decisions that honor both safety needs and human dignity.

Advocating for Responsible Innovation

The ethical integration of technology in Alzheimer's care requires collaboration among stakeholders, including families, caregivers, healthcare providers, and technology developers. Key actions include:

- **Involving Patients and Caregivers**: Include their perspectives in the design and implementation of technologies.

- **Developing Clear Policies**: Establish regulations that prioritize patient rights and ensure accountability for data security.

- **Fostering Transparency**: Encourage open communication about the capabilities and limitations of technological tools.

Closing Thoughts: Balancing Progress with Compassion

Technology has the potential to revolutionize Alzheimer's care, offering solutions that improve safety, diagnosis, and quality of life. However, these advancements must be guided by a strong ethical framework that respects patient autonomy, safeguards privacy, and considers the psychological impact on all involved.

By navigating these challenges responsibly, we can harness the power of innovation while preserving the dignity and humanity of those living with Alzheimer's. This chapter serves as a call to action for families, caregivers, and policymakers to embrace both the opportunities and responsibilities of this new frontier.

Alzheimer's disease not only affects the cognitive abilities of those diagnosed but also places a heavy burden on their families and caregivers to make important legal and ethical decisions. As the disease progresses and individuals lose the ability to express their wishes or make informed choices, caregivers must take on the responsibility of ensuring their loved one's rights, dignity, and well-being are maintained. These decisions often touch upon sensitive issues such as medical treatment, guardianship, financial control, and end-of-life care.

In this chapter, we will explore the key legal and ethical challenges that arise in Alzheimer's care and how families can navigate these difficult decisions. It's essential for caregivers and families to understand these issues early on so that they can plan ahead, respect their loved ones' wishes, and make informed decisions as Alzheimer's advances.

The Importance of Early Legal Planning

The cruelest aspect of Alzheimer's may be its gradual erosion of decision-making capacity, forcing families to assume control over lives that were once fiercely independent. In the early stages of the disease, individuals may still be capable of making their choices about their health, finances, and living arrangements. However, as the disease progresses, they will lose the cognitive ability to make or communicate decisions, leaving these responsibilities to their caregivers.

Early legal planning is crucial for preserving the autonomy and dignity of those diagnosed with Alzheimer's.

By addressing key legal issues early, before cognitive decline sets in, families can ensure that their loved ones' wishes are respected and that the right legal frameworks are in place to protect them. Here are a few important legal tools to consider:

Power of Attorney (POA)

Power of attorney is a legal document that allows an individual to appoint someone they trust to make decisions on their behalf. There are two main types of POA relevant to Alzheimer's care:

Durable Power of Attorney for Health Care: This allows the appointed person (often a family member) to make healthcare decisions for the individual if they become unable to do so.

Durable Power of Attorney for Finances: This gives the appointed person the authority to manage the individual's financial affairs, such as paying bills, managing bank accounts, and handling property.

Establishing a power of attorney while the individual is still able to make informed decisions ensures that they have control over who will be making decisions on their behalf when they can no longer do so. Without the power of attorney, families may need to go through lengthy and costly legal processes to obtain guardianship.

Living Will

A living will is a document that outlines an individual's preferences for medical treatment if they become incapacitated and unable to communicate their wishes. For someone with Alzheimer's, a living will can specify whether they want to receive life-sustaining treatments, such as feeding tubes or mechanical ventilation, if their condition worsens. This document helps alleviate the burden on family members by providing clear guidance on their loved one's end-of-life preferences.

Guardianship and Conservatorship

If legal documents such as power of attorney or living

wills are not in place, families may need to pursue guardianship or conservatorship to manage the affairs of a person with Alzheimer's. Guardianship grants a family member or caregiver legal authority to make personal decisions for the individual, while conservatorship applies to financial decisions. However, these processes can be complex and intrusive, which is why early legal planning is so important.

Ethical Dilemmas in Alzheimer's Care

In addition to legal considerations, families often face difficult ethical dilemmas when caring for a loved one with Alzheimer's. These dilemmas typically revolve around issues of autonomy, quality of life, and balancing the wishes of the individual with the need to ensure their safety and well-being.

Respecting Autonomy vs. Ensuring Safety: One of the most common ethical challenges caregivers face is balancing their loved one's right to make their decisions with the need to keep them safe. In the early stages of Alzheimer's, individuals may still want to live independently, drive, or manage their own finances, but as the disease progresses, these activities can become dangerous.

Families find themselves trapped in impossible dilemmas - forced to choose between honoring their loved one's desire for independence and preventing potential tragedy. For example, taking away the car keys from someone who insists they are still capable of driving can lead to feelings of anger, frustration, and resentment. However, caregivers must weigh these emotional challenges against the risk of harm to their loved one or others.

Quality of Life vs. Length of Life

Another ethical dilemma concerns decisions about medical treatments, particularly in the late stages of Alzheimer's. As the disease progresses and the individual loses the ability to communicate, families must decide whether to pursue aggressive treatments that may prolong life but reduce quality of life.

Many families grapple with whether to continue life-sustaining treatments, such as feeding tubes or resuscitation, when their loved one no longer recognizes them or has no awareness of their surroundings. These decisions can be heart-wrenching, especially when family members have different views on what constitutes a meaningful quality of life.

Truth-Telling and Transparency

A more nuanced ethical issue is whether caregivers should always tell the truth to their loved one with Alzheimer's. In some cases, telling the truth can cause unnecessary distress or confusion. For instance, if a person with Alzheimer's repeatedly asks about a deceased spouse, is it kinder to remind them of the loss each time or to redirect the conversation to something more comforting?

Caregivers often struggle with the ethics of "therapeutic lying," where small deceptions are used to avoid upsetting the person with Alzheimer's. While honesty is generally considered a virtue, caregivers must sometimes weigh the potential harm caused by repeatedly forcing their loved one to confront painful realities.

End-of-Life Care and Decision-Making

As Alzheimer's progresses, many families will face decisions about end-of-life care, including whether to continue certain treatments or transition to palliative or hospice care. These decisions can be emotionally charged, as they involve confronting the inevitable decline of the person they love.

Palliative Care

Palliative care focuses on providing relief from the symptoms and stress of a serious illness, including Alzheimer's. It is designed to improve the quality of life for both the patient and their family by managing symptoms such as pain, anxiety, and difficulty swallowing. Families may consider palliative care when their loved one's condition worsens, allowing them to receive care that prioritizes comfort over curative treatments.

Hospice Care

Hospice care is a type of palliative care provided to individuals who are nearing the end of life. In Alzheimer's care, hospice may be introduced when the individual has advanced to the later stages of the disease, and curative treatments are no longer effective or appropriate. Hospice provides support for both the individual and the family, helping them navigate the emotional, spiritual, and practical aspects of the dying process.

Do Not Resuscitate (DNR) Orders

A DNR order is a legal document that instructs healthcare providers not to perform CPR or other life-saving measures if the individual's heart stops or they stop breathing. For families caring for someone with late-stage Alzheimer's, the decision to implement a DNR order can be one of the most difficult ethical choices they face. While some families may want to do everything possible to prolong life, others may feel that allowing their loved one to pass peacefully is the more compassionate option.

Preparing for Legal and Ethical Challenges

Navigating the legal and ethical challenges of Alzheimer's care can be overwhelming, but there are steps families can take to prepare:

Have Open Conversations Early: Before Alzheimer's progresses, families should have open and honest conversations with their loved ones about their wishes for medical care, end-of-life treatment, and who they want to make decisions on their behalf. These conversations can be difficult but are essential for ensuring that the individual's preferences are respected.

Consult Legal and Medical Professionals: It's important to consult with elder law attorneys and healthcare providers to ensure that all necessary legal documents are in place and that families understand the medical and ethical implications of their decisions. Professionals can help guide familiesthrough complex legal and ethical terrain, providing clarity and support.

Join Support Groups: Many caregivers find it helpful to join support groups where they can discuss legal and ethical dilemmas with others who are going through similar experiences. Support groups provide a safe space to share concerns, receive advice, and learn from others' experiences.

Conclusion

Caring for someone with Alzheimer's is a profound responsibility that extends beyond daily tasks to include difficult legal and ethical decisions. From establishing powers of attorney to making end-of-life care decisions, families must navigate a complex web of choices that impact their loved one's dignity, autonomy, and quality of life.

Early preparation, professional guidance, and compassionate decision-making allow families to become the guardians of both their loved one's physical safety and their lifelong values and preferences. This provides a more hopeful and actionable conclusion.

Alzheimer's may take away a person's ability to make decisions for themselves, but with careful planning and thoughtful consideration, caregivers can ensure that those decisions are made with love and respect.

CHAPTER 12:
THE FUTURE OF ALZHEIMER'S:
HOPE IN MEDICAL DISCOVERIES

"Hope is being able to see that there
is light despite all of the darkness."

-- Desmond Tutu

Alzheimer's stalks its victims like a patient thief, systematically stealing memories, independence, and ultimately, their very sense of self. For families like Claire's, who have spent over a decade witnessing their loved one fade away, the darkness of Alzheimer's can feel overwhelming. Yet even after witnessing Claire's decade-long decline, I have discovered genuine reasons for hope amid the heartbreak.

This hope is found in the laboratories of researchers and the minds of scientists who are determined to understand this disease and ultimately defeat it. In this chapter, we explore the current medical advancements that are shedding light on the path forward, offering hope to those affected by Alzheimer's and their families.

Breakthroughs in Early Diagnosis

One of the most promising areas of Alzheimer's research is the focus on early diagnosis. Early detection of the disease is crucial because it allows for earlier intervention, which could slow progression and improve the quality of life for patients. Researchers have made significant strides in identifying biomarkers - biological indicators that reveal the presence of Alzheimer's before symptoms become severe.

Blood Tests for Alzheimer's

Blood tests for Alzheimer's have evolved from theoretical concepts to clinical reality, offering families a simple, non-invasive way to detect the disease years before cognitive symptoms emerge. These tests measure levels of certain proteins, such as beta-amyloid and tau, which are linked to the development of Alzheimer's. Early research indicates that these blood tests can identify changes in the brain long before memory loss and cognitive decline become evident.

Brain Imaging

Advances in brain imaging technology, such as positron emission tomography (PET) scans and magnetic resonance imaging (MRI), are enabling doctors to see inside the brain and detect the presence of amyloid plaques and tau tangles. These imaging techniques help pinpoint Alzheimer's at an earlier stage, even before significant memory loss occurs. They are also invaluable tools in tracking the progression of the disease and assessing the effectiveness of treatments.

Cognitive Testing

Digital cognitive assessments and apps are being developed to test for early signs of cognitive decline. These tools can monitor memory, attention, and problem-solving abilities over time, helping doctors identify patterns that may signal the onset of Alzheimer's.

Innovative Treatments on the Horizon

Recent advancements in Alzheimer's treatments offer new hope for patients and their families. While scientific progress is promising, it is equally important to understand the practical implications of these therapies, including approval processes, insurance considerations, and guidance for discussing treatment options with healthcare providers.

Anti-Amyloid Therapies: What You Need to Know

Anti-amyloid therapies, such as Aducanumab and Lecanemab, aim to slow cognitive decline by targeting amyloid plaques in the brain. These treatments represent a significant step forward, but they come with important considerations.

Approval Processes

These therapies have undergone rigorous clinical trials to evaluate safety and efficacy. The FDA has granted accelerated approval for some of these drugs, meaning additional data is required to confirm long-term benefits. Patients and caregivers should consult with neurologists specializing in dementia care to determine eligibility for these treatments.

Insurance and Cost Considerations

Medicare and private insurance providers vary in their coverage for anti-amyloid therapies. Out-of-pocket costs can be significant, and financial assistance programs may be available. Patients should inquire about insurance pre-authorization requirements and explore potential cost-saving programs through pharmaceutical manufacturers.

Discussing Treatment with Healthcare Providers

Before starting treatment, patients should undergo comprehensive cognitive assessments and biomarker testing to confirm eligibility. Conversations with doctors should include potential side effects, such as brain swelling or bleeding (ARIA), which require regular monitoring. Patients and caregivers should prepare questions about the expected benefits, risks, and long-term prognosis with treatment.

Beyond Anti-Amyloid Therapies: Emerging

Innovations

Though anti-amyloid treatments dominate headlines, scientists are pursuing multiple parallel paths that attack Alzheimer's from different angles - recognizing that this complex disease likely requires a multi-targeted approach.

Tau-targeting therapies

These aim to address tau protein tangles, another hallmark of Alzheimer's disease. Inflammation reduction treatments

Scientists are exploring ways to minimize neuroinflammation, which contributes to cognitive decline. Gene therapy and personalized medicine

Advancements in genetics may enable tailored treatments based on an individual's risk factors.

Navigating the Future of Alzheimer's Care

With new treatments emerging, families should take a proactive role in advocating for access to innovative care. Stay informed about ongoing clinical trials and potential eligibility for participation. Engage with patient advocacy groups for support and up-to-date information on treatment options. Work closely with medical professionals to evaluate the risks and benefits of new therapies as they become available.

Breakthrough Alzheimer's treatments offer new opportunities, but real-world challenges must be considered. By understanding approval processes, financial implications, and medical guidance, patients and caregivers can make informed decisions about emerging therapies. As research continues to evolve, staying engaged with healthcare professionals and advocacy organizations will be key in navigating the future of Alzheimer's care.

The Role of Technology and AI in Alzheimer's Research

Technology, particularly artificial intelligence (AI), is playing a transformative role in Alzheimer's research and care. AI's ability to analyze vast amounts of data at unprecedented speeds is opening new doors for early detection, personalized treatments, and improved patient outcomes.

AI for Early Diagnosis

AI is being used to analyze brain scans and detect patterns that may indicate Alzheimer's in its earliest stages. AI algorithms can spot subtle changes in brain structure and function that might be missed by the human eye. These advances are helping to diagnose Alzheimer's years before symptoms become apparent, allowing for earlier intervention.

Monitoring Disease Progression

AI-powered tools are also being developed to track the progression of Alzheimer's more precisely. These tools can monitor patients' cognitive and physical changes over time, helping doctors tailor treatments and care plans to each individual's needs. For families like Claire's, this means a better understanding of how the disease is affecting their loved one and more informed decisions about care.

Drug Discovery

AI is accelerating the discovery of new Alzheimer's treatments by analyzing massive datasets from clinical trials and genetic studies. By identifying patterns and connections in this data, AI can predict which drugs are most likely to be effective and which patients may benefit the most. This can drastically reduce the time it takes to develop new treatments and get them to patients.

Wearable Technology

In addition to AI, wearable technology is being integrated into Alzheimer's care. Devices such as smartwatches and biosensors can monitor a patient's physical activity, sleep patterns, and heart rate, providing valuable data that helps track the progression of the disease and alerts caregivers to any sudden changes in behavior or health.

Clinical Trials and the Power of Participation

For families like ours, watching helplessly as Alzheimer's transforms someone we love, clinical trials offer both scientific hope and personal purpose - a chance to reclaim agency in the face of a disease that strips control away. Clinical trials are essential for testing new drugs, treatments, and therapies that could one day change the course of Alzheimer's. Claire's family, like many others, may have considered enrolling in trials as a way to contribute to research that could benefit future generations.

Currently, several clinical trials are underway, investigating everything from anti-amyloid therapies to lifestyle interventions that might reduce the risk of Alzheimer's. Families who choose to participate in clinical trials often feel empowered by contributing to the greater good, knowing that their loved one's experience could help bring new treatments to the world.

A Holistic Approach to Care and Prevention

In addition to these medical breakthroughs, researchers are increasingly recognizing the importance of a holistic approach to Alzheimer's care and prevention. This approach includes:

Diet and Exercise

Studies have shown that a healthy diet, such as the Mediterranean or DASH diet, along with regular physical activity, may reduce the risk of developing Alzheimer's. These lifestyle changes are believed to promote brain health by improving cardiovascular function and reducing inflammation.

Cognitive Stimulation

Engaging in mentally stimulating activities, such as

puzzles, reading, or learning new skills, has been shown to improve cognitive function and potentially delay the onset of Alzheimer's. These activities encourage the brain to form new connections, keeping it resilient against cognitive decline.

Social Interaction

Maintaining social connections and staying engaged with the community is another important aspect of Alzheimer's prevention. Social interaction helps reduce stress and depression, both of which can exacerbate cognitive decline.

The future of Alzheimer's is not without hope. While there is still no cure, the advancements being made in early diagnosis, innovative treatments, and technology provide a glimpse of light in the darkness. For families like Claire's, these breakthroughs represent the possibility of more time to hold onto precious memories, time to connect, and time to care.

Conclusion

Alzheimer's research is advancing at an unprecedented pace, offering a future where the disease's progress can be slowed, its symptoms can be managed more effectively, and, one day, perhaps it will be cured. The hope is that the discoveries being made today will create a better tomorrow for the millions of families affected by this devastating disease.

CHAPTER 13:
BEYOND ONE-SIZE-FITS-ALL:
THE RISE OF PERSONALIZED
ALZHEIMER'S THERAPIES

Imagine a world where Alzheimer's no longer means a slow and painful goodbye; where memories once thought lost could be restored, and families could embrace their loved ones without the fear of fading recognition. The search for effective treatments and, ultimately, a cure for Alzheimer's is one of the most critical medical challenges of our time. While there is still no definitive cure, groundbreaking research is advancing rapidly, offering new hope through promising drug therapies, lifestyle interventions, and innovative treatments like gene therapy and AI-driven diagnostics. The impact of finding an effective treatment would be profound - not only transforming the lives of those diagnosed but also easing the emotional and financial burdens on families and caregivers worldwide. In this chapter, we'll explore the latest advancements in Alzheimer's treatment, shedding light on the strides being made and the hope that lies ahead.

Impact on the Effectiveness of Treatments

Targeted Interventions Based on Genetics

Personalized medicine is no longer just a theoretical concept but an emerging reality that customizes treatments to each person's unique genetic signature, lifestyle patterns, and environmental exposures - offering our first real hope of revolutionizing Alzheimer's care. For instance, researchers have identified several genes that increase the risk of developing Alzheimer's, such as the **APOE ε4 allele**. Patients who carry certain genetic markers may respond better to specific treatments or require tailored interventions to slow disease progression. By identifying these genetic factors early, doctors can implement prevention strategies or personalized drug therapies that might be more effective in delaying the onset or progression of Alzheimer's.

Customized Drug Therapies

The frustrating inconsistency of current Alzheimer's medications stems directly from their development for an 'average patient' who doesn't actually exist - each person's Alzheimer's is as unique as their fingerprint, demanding treatments matched to their specific disease profile. Personalized medicine can change this by tailoring drug therapies to the specific biology of the individual. For example, one patient's Alzheimer's may be more driven by amyloid plaques, while another may be more influenced by tau tangles. Knowing these specifics allows for the development of targeted therapies that directly address the dominant pathology in each patient's brain, potentially leading to better outcomes.

Lifestyle Modifications Based on Risk Profile

In addition to drug therapies, personalized medicine could help tailor lifestyle interventions to an individual's risk factors. For example, a patient whose Alzheimer's risk is increased due to certain cardiovascular markers could benefit from a treatment plan that emphasizes heart health, including dietary changes, exercise, and medications that reduce cholesterol or blood pressure. Personalized recommendations around diet, exercise, and cognitive stimulation could help reduce the risk or slow the progression of Alzheimer's based on each patient's unique risk factors.

Improved Accuracy in Treatment Selection

One of the challenges in treating Alzheimer's is that not all patients respond to the same medications. Personalized medicine would use genetic and molecular data to predict which treatments are most likely to be effective for each individual. This could prevent the time and expense of trying multiple therapies before finding one that works. For example, some patients may respond well to anti-amyloid therapies, while others may benefit more from anti-tau treatments or neuroprotective agents.

Challenges in Developing Personalized Alzheimer's Treatments

Complexity of Alzheimer's as a Disease

One of the biggest challenges in developing personalized medicine for Alzheimer's is the complexity of the disease itself. Alzheimer's is a multifactorial condition, meaning that it is influenced by a wide range of factors, including genetics, lifestyle, environment, and even socioeconomic status. Because the disease manifests differently in different individuals, it is difficult to pinpoint a single treatment approach. For personalized medicine to work effectively, researchers need to deepen their understanding of these complex interactions and develop therapies that can address the full range of factors contributing to Alzheimer's.

High Costs and Access to Treatment

Personalized treatments often come with a high price tag, especially in the early stages of development. While genetic testing costs have plummeted from thousands to hundreds of dollars, the comprehensive analysis, customized treatment formulations, and sophisticated monitoring required for truly personalized care remain prohibitively expensive - threatening to create a two-tiered system where advanced care reaches only the privileged. Ensuring that personalized Alzheimer's treatments are not only effective but also affordable and accessible will be a significant challenge for healthcare systems.

Ethical Concerns and Privacy Issues

As personalized medicine relies heavily on genetic data and other personal health information, there are potential privacy concerns regarding how this data is collected, stored, and used. Patients may be hesitant to participate in genetic testing if they fear their information could be misused by insurers or employers. Our ethical frameworks and privacy regulations, designed for a pre-genomic era, must undergo radical evolution to balance two competing imperatives: protecting intensely personal genetic information from misuse while simultaneously allowing researchers to analyze patterns across thousands of patients to develop effective personalized treatments.

Limited Understanding of Environmental and Lifestyle Factors

While much progress has been made in understanding the genetic factors that contribute to Alzheimer's, the role of environmental and lifestyle factors is still less clear. Personalized medicine relies not only on genetic data but also on understanding how these external factors interact with an individual's biology. More research is needed to identify how specific lifestyle interventions, such as diet, exercise, or stress management, can be tailored to individual patients based on their overall risk profile.

Benefits of Personalized Therapeutic Approaches

Earlier and More Precise Interventions

One of the greatest benefits of personalized medicine is

the potential for earlier and more precise interventions. By identifying genetic markers and risk factors before symptoms even appear, doctors can begin preventive measures earlier, potentially delaying the onset of Alzheimer's. Early interventions, such as lifestyle changes or targeted therapies, may reduce the severity or progression of the disease, giving patients a higher quality of life for longer.

Reduction in Adverse Effects

Personalized medicine could also minimize the risk of adverse drug reactions by ensuring that patients receive treatments suited to their specific biology. For instance, some Alzheimer's patients may be at higher risk for negative side effects from certain medications, while others may metabolize drugs differently based on their genetic profile. Tailoring treatments to each patient's unique biology could improve the safety and tolerability of therapies.

Maximizing Treatment Efficacy

By selecting treatments based on an individual's unique disease profile, personalized medicine has the potential to increase the overall efficacy of Alzheimer's therapies. Patients who receive treatments specifically designed for their form of the disease are more likely to see positive results, reducing frustration for both the patient and their caregivers.

Empowerment for Patients and Families

Personalized medicine also empowers patients and their families by giving them a deeper understanding of the disease and how it affects them personally. With a clearer sense of their genetic risks and personalized treatment options, patients can make more informed decisions about their care. This can provide a greater sense of control and hope in a situation that often feels overwhelming.

The future of Alzheimer's treatment may lie in the promise of personalized medicine. By tailoring therapies to the unique genetic, environmental, and lifestyle factors that influence each individual's experience with Alzheimer's, researchers hope to develop more effective treatments that can slow the progression of the disease or even prevent it. However, realizing the full potential of personalized medicine will require overcoming significant challenges, including the complexity of Alzheimer's, the cost of treatments, and ethical considerations related to data privacy. Despite these hurdles, the move toward personalized therapeutic approaches offers new hope for patients and their families, providing a pathway toward more precise, effective, and compassionate care.

Conclusion

The era of one-size-fits-all Alzheimer's treatment is ending as we enter an age of precision medicine - where understanding your specific genetic vulnerabilities, inflammatory markers, vascular health, and metabolic patterns creates a unique treatment fingerprint that guides intervention from prevention through advanced care.

CHAPTER 14:
WHAT ARE THE ETHICAL
CONSIDERATIONS OF USING
AI AND TECHNOLOGY IN
ALZHEIMER'S CARE?

*"The ethical use of AI in Alzheimer's care
demands a careful balance - leveraging innovation
to enhance lives while fiercely protecting dignity, privacy,
and the humanity of those we aim to support."*
-- Maria L. Ellis

As AI and technology play an increasingly significant role in Alzheimer's care, particularly in early diagnosis, personalized treatment, and disease monitoring, they bring tremendous promise. However, these advancements also raise complex ethical concerns. The use of AI to analyze personal health information, track disease progression, and even predict the onset of Alzheimer's requires careful consideration of privacy, data security, fairness, and patient autonomy. To ensure that AI is used responsibly and ethically in Alzheimer's research and care, specific safeguards must be in place to protect individuals and promote trust in these technologies.

1. Privacy and Data Security Concerns

AI systems in Alzheimer's care rely heavily on vast amounts of personal health data, including genetic information, brain scans, and cognitive assessments. While this data can lead to more accurate diagnoses and better treatment plans, it also creates significant privacy and security risks. Personal health data is incredibly sensitive, and unauthorized access or misuse of this information could have serious consequences for patients, from discrimination in employment or insurance to breaches of medical confidentiality.

The ethical use of AI in Alzheimer's care demands a multi-layered approach to data protection that begins with thorough informed consent - ensuring patients understand how their information will be used and their right to withdraw - and continues through technical safeguards including rigorous anonymization to prevent re-identification, military-grade encryption during storage and transmission, and strict access controls that limit data use to authorized personnel with regular security audits. This comprehensive framework balances the need for rich datasets that improve AI performance against the fundamental right to privacy that remains essential even when cognitive abilities decline.

2. Bias and Fairness in AI Models

Another ethical concern surrounding the use of AI in Alzheimer's care is the potential for bias in AI algorithms. AI systems are trained on large datasets, and if those datasets are not representative of diverse populations, the resulting algorithms may favor certain groups over others. This can lead to disparities in diagnosis, treatment recommendations, and access to care.

For example, AI models trained primarily on data from white Western populations may not perform as well when diagnosing Alzheimer's in individuals from different ethnic backgrounds or regions. This could result in delayed or inaccurate diagnoses for underrepresented groups, exacerbating existing healthcare inequalities.

To address fairness concerns, several safeguards should be considered:

Diverse Datasets

AI models should be trained on datasets that are diverse and representative of the broader population. This includes data from individuals of different ethnicities, genders, socioeconomic backgrounds, and geographic locations. Ensuring diversity in the data will make AI systems more equitable and improve their accuracy for all patients.

Bias Auditing

AI models should undergo regular audits to check for potential biases. These audits can help identify areas where the algorithm may be favoring one group over another and allow developers to adjust the model to ensure fairness.

Transparency

AI systems should be designed to be transparent in how they reach conclusions, so healthcare providers and patients can understand how decisions are made. This transparency builds trust and allows for accountability if biases are discovered.

3. Autonomy and Patient Consent

The use of AI in Alzheimer's care also raises questions about patient autonomy and decision-making. Alzheimer's patients, particularly those in the later stages of the disease, may lose the ability to make informed decisions about their care. While AI can help caregivers make more informed decisions on behalf of their loved ones, there is a risk that patients may feel their autonomy is being undermined if decisions are driven solely by algorithmic recommendations.

To ensure patient autonomy is respected, safeguards should include:

Shared Decision-Making

AI should support, not replace, human decision-making in Alzheimer's care. Doctors, patients, and their families should be involved in the decision-making process, using AI as a tool to provide insights rather than allowing it to dictate care. AI should enhance the ability to make informed choices rather than limit patient autonomy.

Regular Review of AI Recommendations

AI-generated recommendations should be regularly reviewed by healthcare professionals to ensure they align with the patient's preferences and evolving needs. If a patient or their family disagrees with an AI-based recommendation, there should be a clear process for overriding the AI decision in favor of human judgment.

Advanced Directives

In cases where patients are no longer able to make decisions due to cognitive decline, AI should be used in conjunction with the patient's previously expressed wishes, such as those outlined in advance directives. These directives should guide the use of AI in making decisions about treatments, interventions, and end-of-life care.

4. Ownership of Data and Results

One key question in AI-driven Alzheimer's care is **who owns the data** and the results generated by AI algorithms. Since patient data is used to train AI models and create personalized care plans, questions of ownership and control over this information are critical.

Patient Control Over Data

Patients should retain ownership of their health data and have the right to determine how it is used. If an AI system uses their data for research purposes, patients should be informed and have the option to consent or decline. Additionally, patients should be able to access the insights or results that AI generates about their condition.

Sharing Research Findings

If AI systems identify new patterns in Alzheimer's that could benefit the broader community, there should be clear guidelines on how these findings are shared with the scientific community while still protecting patient privacy. Research derived from AI should contribute to the greater good, but this must be balanced with respecting individual privacy rights.

5. Accountability and Transparency

When AI is used to make recommendations for diagnosis or treatment, it is important to determine who is responsible for those decisions. If an AI system makes a mistake, leading to a misdiagnosis or ineffective treatment, who is held accountable - the developers of the AI, the healthcare providers who relied on it, or the institution that deployed it?

Clear Accountability Structures

There must be clear accountability structures in place that define who is responsible for the outcomes of AI-driven decisions. AI should be viewed as a tool that assists healthcare professionals rather than an independent decision-maker. Healthcare providers should remain responsible for reviewing and approving AI recommendations.

Transparency in AI Systems

AI systems should be designed with transparency in mind, meaning healthcare providers and patients should understand how the AI arrived at a particular decision or recommendation. This "explainability" is crucial for building trust and ensuring that decisions made by AI can be scrutinized and adjusted if necessary.

6. The Potential for Over-Reliance on AI

While AI has tremendous potential, there is a risk that healthcare providers may become overly reliant on AI systems, leading to a reduction in human judgment and empathy in patient care. Alzheimer's patients, in particular, require compassionate, person-centered care that cannot be fully replaced by technology.

Balanced Use of AI

AI should be used to complement human judgment, not replace it. Caregivers and healthcare professionals must continue to exercise their clinical expertise and empathy in decision-making. The goal of AI should be to enhance the quality of care, providing data-driven insights while still prioritizing human connections and interactions in the care of Alzheimer's patients.

AI and technology have the potential to significantly improve Alzheimer's care, from early diagnosis to personalized treatment. However, these advancements come with ethical challenges that must be addressed to ensure patient safety, privacy, and autonomy. Safeguards such as strong data protection, transparency, bias auditing, and ensuring accountability will help build trust in AI systems and promote their responsible use in Alzheimer's research and care. Ultimately, AI should be a tool that supports both patients and caregivers, enhancing care while respecting the dignity and rights of those living with Alzheimer's.

What Role Do Lifestyle Interventions Play Alongside Medical Advancements in Alzheimer's Prevention?

As our understanding of Alzheimer's disease continues to evolve, one of the most promising areas of research focuses on the role of **lifestyle interventions** - such as diet, exercise, and mental stimulation - in preventing or delaying the onset of the disease. While medical advancements, including new drugs and diagnostic tools, play a crucial role in treating Alzheimer's, lifestyle factors are increasingly recognized as key components in brain health. When combined with medical treatments, these interventions may not only enhance cognitive function but also potentially reduce the need for certain medications or delay the disease's progression.

The Power of Diet in Alzheimer's Prevention

Emerging research suggests that **diet** can have a

profound effect on brain health and may reduce the risk of Alzheimer's. Two diets, in particular, have gained attention for their neuroprotective benefits: the **Mediterranean diet** and the **DASH (Dietary Approaches to Stop Hypertension) diet**. Both are rich in vegetables, fruits, whole grains, lean proteins (especially fish), nuts, and healthy fats, such as olive oil. These diets are also low in red meat, processed foods, and refined sugars, which are linked to increased inflammation and oxidative stress in the brain.

The **Mediterranean-DASH Diet Intervention for Neurodegenerative Delay (MIND)** diet is a hybrid of the two and is specifically designed to support brain health. Studies have shown that people who adhere to the MIND diet may have a lower risk of developing Alzheimer's disease, with some research suggesting a delay in the onset of cognitive decline by up to 7.5 years. The MIND diet emphasizes leafy green vegetables, berries, and omega-3-rich fish, all of which are known to promote brain health.

Integrating Diet with Medical Treatments

For individuals at risk of Alzheimer's, adopting a brain-healthy diet can complement medical treatments aimed at slowing cognitive decline. By reducing inflammation and improving cardiovascular health, a healthy diet may support the effectiveness of medications designed to protect neurons or reduce amyloid plaque buildup.

In some cases, lifestyle changes, including diet, may reduce the need for certain medications, particularly those aimed at managing cardiovascular risk factors, such as high blood pressure and cholesterol - conditions linked to cognitive decline.

Exercise as a Protective Factor for the Brain

Regular **physical exercise** is another powerful intervention for Alzheimer's prevention. Physical activity boosts blood flow to the brain, promotes the growth of new neurons, and reduces inflammation - all factors that help protect against cognitive decline. Studies show that regular aerobic exercise (such as walking, swimming, or cycling) can improve memory, attention, and problem-solving skills, even in older adults. Exercise has also been shown to reduce the levels of beta-amyloid and tau proteins, which are associated with Alzheimer's.

Exercise not only enhances physical health but also improves **neuroplasticity**, the brain's ability to form new neural connections. This is particularly important for people at risk of Alzheimer's, as it helps build cognitive resilience, making the brain better equipped to resist damage from neurodegenerative diseases.

Integrating Exercise with Medical Treatments

Exercise could be a vital **adjunct to drug therapy** for Alzheimer's. For example, individuals undergoing pharmacological treatment to slow cognitive decline could experience greater benefits when combining their medications with regular physical activity. This is because exercise stimulates brain-derived neurotrophic factor (BDNF), a protein that supports the survival and growth of neurons, enhancing the brain's ability to repair itself.

Additionally, exercise can help manage conditions like hypertension and diabetes, which are linked to an increased risk of Alzheimer's, potentially reducing the need for medications targeting these conditions.

Mental Stimulation and Cognitive Health

Cognitive decline is not only about memory loss but also about the loss of flexibility in thinking and problem-solving. Engaging in **mentally stimulating activities** - such as learning new skills, solving puzzles, playing musical instruments, or even socializing - can help preserve cognitive function and delay the onset of Alzheimer's.

Activities that challenge the brain promote **cognitive reserve**, which refers to the brain's ability to compensate for damage caused by Alzheimer's or other neurological conditions. Research shows that individuals with higher levels of education or those who engage in lifelong learning are less likely to experience severe cognitive decline, even if they have Alzheimer's pathology in their brains. Mental stimulation builds stronger neural networks that can continue to function despite age-related damage.

Integrating Mental Stimulation with Medical Treatments

Combining medical treatments with cognitive training programs could enhance the benefits of pharmacological interventions. For instance, patients taking memory-enhancing drugs may achieve better results if they also engage in regular mental exercises designed to improve memory, attention, and executive functioning.

Digital tools and apps that offer brain-training exercises are becoming more popular, and they could be prescribed alongside medical treatments to keep the brain engaged and active. Such tools might also help doctors monitor cognitive changes in real time, providing valuable feedback for adjusting medications or therapies.

Social Engagement and Mental Well-Being

Maintaining **social connections** is another essential aspect of Alzheimer's prevention. Social isolation and loneliness have been linked to an increased risk of Alzheimer's and other forms of dementia. In contrast, staying socially active can help reduce stress, depression, and anxiety, all of which negatively impact brain health. Being part of a community, whether through volunteer work, social clubs, or simply staying connected with friends and family, stimulates mental engagement and provides emotional support.

Integrating Social Interaction with Medical Treatments

Social engagement can enhance the emotional and psychological well-being of Alzheimer's patients, improving their response to medical treatments. For example, patients who are involved in social activities may experience better mood regulation and motivation, which can help them adhere to treatment plans and maintain a higher quality of life.

Alzheimer's support groups, both for patients and caregivers, offer a dual benefit: they provide emotional support while also serving as a platform for sharing information on lifestyle interventions, new treatments, and coping strategies. Social connections within these groups can reduce the stress of caregiving and help families implement holistic approaches to care.

Could Preventive Measures Reduce the Need for Medications or Delay the Onset of Alzheimer's?

Lifestyle interventions, particularly when implemented early, have the potential to **delay the onset of Alzheimer's** or reduce the severity of its progression. By addressing modifiable risk factors - such as diet, exercise, and mental stimulation - individuals can build cognitive resilience, which may delay the need for medications or reduce their dependency on them.

In some cases, lifestyle changes could delay the transition from mild cognitive impairment (MCI) to Alzheimer's, giving individuals more years of independence before they require medical treatment. For example, a person with a family history of Alzheimer's who adopts a brain-healthy lifestyle at age fifty might delay cognitive decline by several years, potentially avoiding or reducing the need for memory-enhancing drugs until much later in life.

Furthermore, preventive lifestyle interventions could reduce the burden on healthcare systems by lowering the prevalence of Alzheimer's, as fewer people may require intensive treatments or long-term care. For families, this means a reduced emotional and financial burden, as lifestyle-based prevention could delay the need for specialized Alzheimer's care or costly medications.

While medical advancements continue to bring hope for new treatments and diagnostic tools, lifestyle interventions - such as a healthy diet, regular exercise, mental stimulation, and social engagement - play an equally important role in Alzheimer's prevention. These lifestyle factors not only support brain health but also complement medical treatments by enhancing their effectiveness, reducing the need for certain medications, and potentially delaying the onset of Alzheimer's.

By integrating lifestyle changes with medical therapies, healthcare providers can offer a more **holistic approach** to Alzheimer's care - one that not only treats the disease but also empowers individuals and families to take proactive steps in maintaining cognitive health and quality of life.

How Can Clinical Trials Be Made More Accessible to Families Dealing with Alzheimer's?

Clinical trials play a crucial role in the development of new treatments and therapies for Alzheimer's disease. They offer patients and caregivers a sense of hope, with the potential to benefit not only themselves but future generations. However, despite the importance of these trials, many families dealing with Alzheimer's find it difficult to participate due to several barriers, including geographic location, time constraints, and financial challenges. Making clinical trials more accessible is essential to ensure diverse participation and speed up the development of effective treatments.

Overcoming Geographic Barriers

One of the most significant barriers to clinical trial participation is the **location** of the trial sites. Many Alzheimer's clinical trials are conducted at major medical research centers, which are often located in large cities. For families living in rural or suburban areas, the need to travel long distances can be a major obstacle, especially when managing the care of a loved one with Alzheimer's.

Solutions to Improve Access

Decentralized Clinical Trials (DCTs): Advances in technology are enabling **decentralized clinical** trials, which allow participants to be monitored and treated from home rather than requiring frequent visits to a research center. This model leverages telemedicine, remote monitoring devices, and online data collection, making it easier for families to participate without the need to travel. Decentralized trials can also include home visits from healthcare professionals, ensuring that participants still receive high-quality care while remaining in a familiar environment.

Satellite Sites and Regional Partnerships: Expanding clinical trials to **satellite sites** in smaller hospitals, local clinics, or community health centers can bring trials closer to participants. By partnering with regional healthcare providers, research institutions can widen their geographic reach and involve a more diverse population in Alzheimer's research.

Transportation Assistance: Some trial sponsors and organizations are beginning to offer **transportation assistance** for families who need help traveling to trial sites. Providing transportation vouchers or reimbursing travel expenses can ease the burden of accessing clinical trials for those who live further away.

Addressing Time and Caregiving Constraints

Caring for someone with Alzheimer's is already a full-time job for many families, and the additional time commitment required for clinical trial participation can feel overwhelming. Frequent site visits, tests, and assessments can take time away from caregiving responsibilities, making it difficult for families to balance trial participation with their daily lives.

Solutions to Reduce the Time Burden

Flexible Trial Scheduling: Offering **flexible scheduling** for trial-related appointments, including evening or weekend hours, can make it easier for caregivers and patients to participate. Some trials are beginning to adopt more family-friendly schedules to accommodate the needs of caregivers who may work or have other responsibilities.

At-Home Care Services: For trials that do require

onsite participation, providing **at-home care services** for the Alzheimer's patient during the caregiver's absence can help. By covering the cost of temporary respite care, clinical trial sponsors can reduce the pressure on caregivers and encourage more families to participate.

Shortened Trial Visits: Streamlining clinical trial protocols to minimize the number of on-site visits or reduce the duration of each visit can also help. By using **digital tools** to collect data remotely, trials can limit the need for lengthy in-person assessments, allowing participants to contribute without significant disruptions to their routines.

Reducing Financial Barriers

The **financial burden** of Alzheimer's care is already significant for many families, and participation in clinical trials can add additional costs, including travel, lodging, and missed workdays. While many clinical trials cover the cost of treatments and tests, families are often left to shoulder other expenses that may make participation financially unfeasible.

Solutions to Ease Financial Concerns

Financial Compensation: Offering **financial compensation** to participants can help offset the cost of travel, lodging, or lost income due to missed work. While compensation is often provided in clinical trials, ensuring that it is sufficient to cover all out-of-pocket expenses is crucial to making trials more accessible to low- and middle-income families.

Reimbursement for Care-Related Costs: In addition to compensating for travel or missed work, trials can also offer **reimbursement for caregiving expenses**, such as hiring professional caregivers to assist with the patient during trial participation.

Collaborating with Insurance Providers: In some cases, families may hesitate to join a trial because they fear certain costs (such as related treatments or emergency care) won't be covered by insurance. Collaborating with insurance providers to **guarantee coverage** for trial-related medical needs can give families peace of mind and encourage participation.

Increasing Awareness and Communication About Clinical Trials

Many families are simply unaware that clinical trials are an option or may not know how to find trials that are relevant to their loved one's condition. Lack of information and poor communication between healthcare providers and patients about ongoing trials can limit participation, particularly in underrepresented communities.

What Are the Challenges in Bringing New Alzheimer's Drugs and Treatments from Research to Widespread Use?

The journey from laboratory discovery to widely available Alzheimer's treatments involve formidable obstacles that delay critical therapies from reaching patients. Despite research breakthroughs, the path to market is hindered by regulatory hurdles, financial risks, and accessibility issues that require collaborative solutions between pharmaceutical companies, governments, and regulatory agencies.

The drug development timeline for Alzheimer's treatments typically spans over a decade and costs approximately $2.6 billion. This process begins with preclinical testing, where many promising compounds fail due to the brain's complexity making animal results poor predictors of human outcomes. Clinical trials then progress through three increasingly rigorous phases, with Alzheimer's trials presenting unique difficulties due to the disease's slow progression requiring lengthy studies and challenging participant recruitment criteria. Even after promising early results, many treatments fail in Phase 3, magnifying costs and development timelines.

Regulatory approval presents another significant barrier. Agencies like the FDA and EMA rightfully demand extensive safety and efficacy evidence, which is particularly crucial for vulnerable Alzheimer's patients. However, the disease's lack of definitive biomarkers complicates demonstrating treatment effectiveness, often leading to approval delays or rejections. Post-approval monitoring requirements add further complexity and expense for pharmaceutical companies.

The financial landscape for Alzheimer's drug development is exceptionally risky. With historic failure rates approaching 99.6 percent between 2002 and 2012, many companies have scaled back Alzheimer's research despite the massive unmet need. Even successfully approved drugs face commercial challenges, including pricing structures, insurance reimbursement, and market competition. These financial uncertainties discourage investment in a field desperately needing innovation.

Accelerating treatment development requires enhanced collaboration. Fast-track regulatory designations for serious unmet needs like Alzheimer's can significantly reduce time to market. Public-private partnerships such as the Accelerating Medicines Partnership pool resources and expertise, while open-access data sharing from both successful and failed trials prevents duplicated efforts and builds collective knowledge.

Even after approval, ensuring treatment accessibility remains challenging. New Alzheimer's drugs often carry premium prices to recover R&D investments, placing them beyond reach for many patients, especially those on fixed incomes. Geographical and socioeconomic disparities in treatment availability further complicate equitable distribution. Value-based pricing models that link cost to demonstrated effectiveness offer one potential solution that balances innovation incentives with accessibility needs.

Despite these challenges, collaborative efforts can overcome these obstacles. By streamlining approval processes, sharing financial risks through innovative funding models, and prioritizing affordable access, we can accelerate the development of treatments that offer hope to millions of families affected by Alzheimer's. Though the journey remains difficult, the potential to transform lives makes this pursuit essential.

How Might Global Collaboration Accelerate Alzheimer's Research and Treatment Development?

Alzheimer's disease is a global public health challenge that affects millions of people across every continent. Despite its prevalence, the path to effective treatments and cures has been slow and fraught with setbacks. However, global collaboration offers a way to accelerate Alzheimer's research by bringing together diverse expertise, expanding research opportunities, and pooling resources. By fostering international partnerships and promoting data sharing across borders, researchers can speed up the discovery of new treatments, learn from diverse populations, and tackle this complex disease from multiple angles.

1. The Importance of Global Collaboration in Alzheimer's Research

Alzheimer's disease doesn't recognize borders, and neither should the search for a cure. Global collaboration allows researchers to combine efforts and share knowledge, which can lead to more significant breakthroughs in a shorter period. By working together, countries can:

Expand Research Opportunities

Collaboration enables researchers to tap into larger and more diverse populations for clinical trials, which is essential for understanding how Alzheimer's affects different groups and how treatments work across various genetic and environmental contexts.

Pool Resources and Expertise

International partnerships allow for the sharing of financial resources, advanced technologies, and specialized expertise that may not be available in individual countries. This pooling of resources helps reduce duplication of efforts and maximizes the impact of research funding.

Accelerate Data Collection and Analysis

By sharing data across borders, researchers can gather and analyze information more quickly. This speeds up the research process, allowing scientists to identify patterns and potential treatments sooner.

2. Data Sharing and Standardization Across Borders

One of the most significant benefits of global collaboration is the ability to share data. Alzheimer's research generates vast amounts of data, from genetic information and brain imaging to clinical trial results. Sharing this data internationally allows for larger, more comprehensive studies and helps researchers identify trends that may be missed in smaller, localized studies.

Key Steps to Accelerate Data Sharing

- **Creating Global Databases**: Establishing centralized, global databases that store clinical trial data, genetic information, and brain imaging results allows researchers to access and analyze data from diverse populations. Examples include the Global Alzheimer's Association Interactive Network (GAAIN), which allows researchers worldwide to share and analyze Alzheimer's data, and the Alzheimer's Disease Neuroimaging Initiative (ADNI), which provides access to imaging data from thousands of Alzheimer's patients across the globe.

- **Standardizing Data Collection**: For international collaboration to be effective, data must be collected in a standardized way. This ensures that data from different countries can be accurately compared and analyzed. Creating global protocols for clinical trials, imaging techniques, and cognitive assessments can help ensure consistency across research sites.

3. Examples of Successful Global Partnerships in Alzheimer's Research

Several global partnerships have already demonstrated the power of international collaboration in advancing Alzheimer's research. These initiatives show how pooling resources, expertise, and data can accelerate the discovery of new treatments and improve our understanding of the disease.

The World Wide Alzheimer's Disease Neuroimaging Initiative (WW-ADNI)

Building on the success of the U.S.-based ADNI, WW-ADNI is a global collaboration involving researchers from North America, Europe, Japan, Australia, and China. Its goal is to study how Alzheimer's develops by tracking changes in the brain using neuroimaging, biomarkers, and clinical assessments. By comparing data across different countries, researchers can better understand how Alzheimer's progresses in different populations and identify potential early indicators of the disease. This initiative has led to important discoveries about Alzheimer's biomarkers and has accelerated the development of diagnostic tools.

The European Prevention of Alzheimer's Dementia (EPAD) Initiative

EPAD is a public-private partnership funded by the European Union that aims to improve the design of clinical trials for Alzheimer's disease. It brings together academic institutions, pharmaceutical companies, and public organizations from across Europe to develop new strategies for early diagnosis and prevention. EPAD's innovative adaptive trial platform allows for more efficient clinical trials by testing multiple treatments simultaneously in a large cohort of at-risk individuals. This flexible approach reduces the time and cost of testing potential therapies and increases the chances of finding effective treatments.

The Dementia Discovery Fund (DDF)

The DDF is a global venture capital fund focused on financing innovative Alzheimer's research. Established by major pharmaceutical companies, charitable foundations, and government entities, the fund invests in early-stage research with the potential to transform dementia treatment. By bringing together resources from around the world, the DDF supports cutting-edge research into new drug targets, diagnostic tools, and therapies. One of the key benefits of the DDF is that it enables researchers to take bold, high-risk approaches that might not receive traditional funding.

Joint Programming Initiative on Neurodegenerative Disease Research (JPND)

The JPND is Europe's largest collaborative research effort aimed at tackling neurodegenerative diseases, including Alzheimer's. It brings together thirty member countries to align research priorities, pool funding, and share data. One of JPND's key achievements is the development of a common research strategy, which ensures that efforts are coordinated and that resources are directed toward the most promising areas of research. JPND also fosters partnerships with non-European countries to expand the scope of its research.

4. The Role of International Clinical Trials

International clinical trials are critical for developing Alzheimer's treatments that work across diverse populations. Conducting trials in multiple countries ensures that drugs are effective in people with different genetic backgrounds, lifestyles, and environmental exposures. Global trials can also accelerate the recruitment process, allowing researchers to reach the required number of participants more quickly.

Benefits of International Clinical Trials

- **Diversity of Participants**: Alzheimer's research often suffers from a lack of diversity in clinical trials, with many studies conducted primarily on Western populations. International trials help ensure that new treatments are tested on people from various ethnicities and regions, which is crucial for understanding how these treatments work globally.

- **Faster Recruitment**: By expanding the pool of potential participants across multiple countries, international trials can overcome one of the biggest challenges in Alzheimer's research: recruiting enough patients to generate meaningful results. Faster recruitment shortens the overall time it takes to complete a trial and bring treatment to market.

- **Regulatory Harmonization**: One challenge in conducting international trials is navigating different regulatory environments. However, efforts to harmonize regulatory requirements across countries, such as through the International Council for Harmonization of Technical Requirements for Pharmaceuticals for Human Use (ICH), can make it easier to run clinical trials across borders.

5. The Future of Global Collaboration in Alzheimer's Research

Looking ahead, the future of global collaboration in Alzheimer's research will likely involve even greater integration of advanced technologies, such as artificial intelligence (AI) and machine learning, to analyze vast datasets from around the world. AI can help researchers identify patterns in complex datasets that would be difficult or impossible to detect manually, accelerating the discovery of new biomarkers and treatment targets.

Key Priorities for Future Collaboration

- **Expanding Global Research Networks**: Building on existing partnerships, researchers can continue to expand global research networks to include more countries, particularly those in low- and middle-income regions where Alzheimer's research is currently limited. This will increase the diversity of the research and provide new insights into how Alzheimer's develops in different populations.

- **Funding and Resource Sharing**: Governments, philanthropic organizations, and private companies must continue to collaborate to provide the necessary funding for large-scale, international research projects. Resource sharing, such as access to specialized imaging equipment or genetic databases, will help make the most of the available funding and ensure that research efforts are coordinated.

- **Public Engagement and Education**: To facilitate global collaboration, it's essential to engage the public and raise awareness about the importance of participating in Alzheimer's research. International campaigns to educate people about clinical trials, genetic studies, and preventive measures can increase participation and support from diverse communities.

Global collaboration is key to accelerating Alzheimer's research and treatment development. By pooling resources, sharing data, and working together across borders, researchers can overcome the challenges of Alzheimer's more effectively and efficiently. Successful global partnerships, such as the WW-ADNI, EPAD, and the DDF, demonstrate the power of international collaboration in advancing our understanding of Alzheimer's and developing new treatments. As Alzheimer's continues to affect millions of people worldwide, fostering these global connections will be essential in the search for a cure.

What Role Does Public Awareness Play in Driving Funding and Support for Alzheimer's Research?

Alzheimer's disease is one of the most significant health challenges of our time, but it remains underfunded compared to other major diseases. To accelerate progress in Alzheimer's research, substantial funding is required - not just from governments and pharmaceutical companies, but also from private donations, foundations, and grassroots efforts. Public awareness campaigns play a crucial role in raising the necessary funds and building political support for Alzheimer's research. These campaigns inform people about the devastating effects of the disease, the urgent need for more research, and the ways individuals can get involved in supporting the cause. Through advocacy, patients and their families have the power to shape public policy, direct more funding to research, and accelerate the development of treatments.

The Importance of Public Awareness in Alzheimer's Research Funding

Public awareness is vital to securing the funding needed for Alzheimer's research. When people are informed about the scale of the Alzheimer's crisis - both in terms of the number of people affected and the emotional, financial, and social toll of the disease - they are more likely to donate to research initiatives and advocate for greater government support.

Public awareness campaigns have several important functions:

- **Increasing Visibility of the Disease**: Alzheimer's is often misunderstood or seen as an inevitable part of aging rather than a disease that can be treated or cured. Public awareness helps educate the general public about the seriousness of the disease and the urgent need for research.

- **Building Political Will**: Governments are more likely to allocate funds for Alzheimer's research when there is strong public demand. Awareness campaigns can mobilize voters to pressure politicians to prioritize Alzheimer's funding in national healthcare and research budgets.

- **Attracting Private Donations**: Many Alzheimer's research initiatives are funded by private donations. Well-executed public awareness campaigns can inspire individuals, philanthropists, and corporations to contribute to Alzheimer's research efforts.

Successful Examples of Advocacy Driving Alzheimer's Research Funding

Several advocacy groups and awareness campaigns have successfully driven substantial funding and political support for Alzheimer's research. Here are a few notable examples:

The Alzheimer's Association and the Walk to End Alzheimer's

One of the most influential organizations in Alzheimer's advocacy is the **Alzheimer's Association**, which has raised billions of dollars for research and support services through its nationwide events, including the Walk to End Alzheimer's. This annual event, which takes place in hundreds of communities across the United States, raises both awareness and funds for Alzheimer's research. Participants come together to walk in honor of those affected by the disease, creating a powerful sense of solidarity and purpose. The funds raised from these events have been instrumental in supporting cutting-edge research projects, care services, and public education efforts.

The Alzheimer's Impact Movement (AIM)

The **Alzheimer's Impact Movement (AIM)**, an advocacy arm of the Alzheimer's Association, focuses specifically on influencing public policy and increasing government funding for Alzheimer's research. AIM works with legislators to ensure that Alzheimer's is a priority on the national political agenda. Thanks to their efforts, the U.S. Congress has significantly increased funding for Alzheimer's research at the National Institutes of Health (NIH). In fact, federal funding for Alzheimer's research has grown from $631 million in 2015 to over $3.5 billion in 2023, making it one of the most well-funded areas of medical research in the U.S. This increase is largely due to the persistent efforts of AIM and other advocacy groups, which have worked tirelessly to raise awareness and secure political support.

World Alzheimer's Month

Every September, Alzheimer's Month is observed globally to raise awareness about Alzheimer's and dementia. Organized by Alzheimer's Disease International (ADI), this campaign reaches millions of people and encourages countries to make Alzheimer's a public health priority. Governments, businesses, and non-governmental organizations participate in the campaign, helping to spread awareness, reduce stigma, and promote the need for more research. The campaign also encourages people to participate in fundraising events or advocate for more support for those affected by the disease. World Alzheimer's Month has become a key driver for both local and international funding for Alzheimer's research and care.

The Dementia Friends Initiative

Started in the UK, the Dementia Friends initiative encourages people to become "Dementia Friends" by learning more about Alzheimer's and how to support those living with dementia. This movement has spread to more than fifty countries, reaching millions of people globally. The initiative emphasizes that even small actions - like volunteering, participating in advocacy, or fundraising - can make a big difference. This grassroots movement has raised substantial funds for dementia research and has helped build a strong network of advocates.

How Patients and Families Can Become Advocates for Change

Patients, caregivers, and families affected by Alzheimer's are some of the most powerful advocates for change. Their firsthand experiences with the disease provide compelling narratives that can motivate others to get involved and encourage politicians to take action. Here are several ways that families and individuals can advocate for Alzheimer's research and support:

Share Their Story

Personal stories are often the most impactful tools in advocacy. By sharing their experiences with Alzheimer's - whether through social media, local newspapers, or public speaking events - patients and families can raise awareness about the challenges of the disease. These stories put a human face on the statistics, helping to illustrate the urgent need for funding and research.

Participate in Advocacy Days

Many Alzheimer's organizations host advocacy days, where patients, caregivers, and supporters meet with lawmakers to discuss Alzheimer's research and funding. These events give families the opportunity to directly influence public policy by sharing their experiences with decision-makers. For example, the Alzheimer's Association's Advocacy Forum in Washington, D.C., brings together thousands of advocates from across the U.S. to meet with members of Congress and push for increased research funding.

Get Involved with Local and National Organizations

Families can join local Alzheimer's organizations or chapters of national groups like the Alzheimer's Association to participate in fundraising events, advocacy efforts, and awareness campaigns. Joining forces with these groups amplifies their voices and helps create a unified front in the fight against Alzheimer's.

Fundraising for Research

Patients and their families can play a critical role in funding Alzheimer's research by organizing or participating in fundraising events. Activities like walks, marathons, charity dinners, and online crowdfunding campaigns can raise significant amounts of money. Families can also set up memorial funds or tribute donations in honor of loved ones affected by the disease.

Engage in Social Media Campaigns

Social media is a powerful tool for raising awareness and mobilizing support. By participating in online campaigns - such as sharing facts about Alzheimer's, using relevant hashtags, or encouraging donations - families can reach a wider audience. Platforms like Facebook, Twitter, and Instagram allow advocates to connect with others who are passionate about finding a cure for Alzheimer's and to share their stories with a global audience.

Conclusion

Families can advocate for increased government funding by contacting their elected officials and urging them to prioritize Alzheimer's research in national budgets. Writing letters, making phone calls, and attending town hall meetings are effective ways to make their voices heard. Organizations like the Alzheimer's Association provide resources and templates to help families advocate for research funding and policy changes.

CHAPTER 15:
HOW ARE EMERGING THERAPIES, LIKE GENE EDITING OR STEM CELL TREATMENTS, BEING EXPLORED FOR ALZHEIMER'S CARE?

"Emerging therapies like gene editing and stem cell treatments hold the promise to not only treat Alzheimer's but to redefine what is possible in restoring memory, identity, and the essence of life itself."
-- Maria L. Ellis

Alzheimer's disease has long posed a formidable challenge to researchers due to its complex and multifactorial nature. While current treatments focus on managing symptoms and slowing cognitive decline, emerging fields such as gene editing and stem cell therapy offer exciting new possibilities for addressing the underlying causes of the disease. These cutting-edge therapies have the potential to change the landscape of Alzheimer's care by targeting the genetic and cellular mechanisms that drive neurodegeneration. Although still in the early stages of development, these therapies hold promises for not only slowing the progression of Alzheimer's but potentially preventing or even reversing its effects in the future.

How Are Emerging Therapies, Like Gene Editing or Stem Cell Treatments, Being Explored

for Alzheimer's Care?

Alzheimer's disease has long posed a formidable challenge to researchers due to its complex and multifactorial nature. While current treatments focus on managing symptoms and slowing cognitive decline, emerging fields such as gene editing and stem cell therapy offer exciting new possibilities for addressing the underlying causes of the disease. These cutting-edge therapies have the potential to change the landscape of Alzheimer's care by targeting the genetic and cellular mechanisms that drive neurodegeneration. Although still in the early stages of development, these therapies hold promise for not only slowing the progression of Alzheimer's but potentially preventing or even reversing its effects in the future.

Gene Editing: Rewriting the Genetic Code

Gene editing is a groundbreaking approach that aims to modify or correct genetic mutations associated with diseases, including Alzheimer's. The development of precise gene-editing technologies, such as **CRISPR-Cas9**, has opened new doors for Alzheimer's research, enabling scientists to directly target and alter specific genes linked to the disease.

How Gene Editing Works

CRISPR-Cas9 technology acts like molecular scissors, allowing researchers to cut DNA at specific points in the genome. Once the DNA is cut, scientists can either disable harmful genes, repair mutations, or introduce new genetic material that can protect against disease. In the context of Alzheimer's, CRISPR can be used to target genes associated with the production of proteins that contribute to neurodegeneration, such as amyloid-beta and tau.

Gene Editing in Alzheimer's Research

One of the most well-known genetic risk factors for Alzheimer's is the APOE ε4 allele. People who carry this variant of the APOE gene are at a significantly higher risk of developing Alzheimer's, particularly in later life. Gene-editing technologies like CRISPR could potentially be used to either turn off the APOE ε4 gene or replace it with a less harmful variant, such as APOE ε2, which is associated with a reduced risk of Alzheimer's.

Early-stage research has shown promising results in using CRISPR to reduce the levels of amyloid-beta and tau, the proteins that accumulate in the brains of people with Alzheimer's. By editing genes responsible for the production of these proteins, scientists hope to reduce or eliminate the toxic build-up of amyloid plaques and tau tangles, which are hallmarks of the disease.

Challenges and Potential of Gene Editing

While gene editing holds great promise, there are significant challenges to overcome before it can become a viable treatment for Alzheimer's. One concern is the **safety and precision** of gene editing. Off-target effects, where unintended genes are edited, could lead to unintended consequences, including the risk of introducing new mutations. Ensuring that CRISPR can accurately and safely target specific genes in the brain is a key hurdle that researchers are actively working to address.

Despite these challenges, the potential of gene editing in Alzheimer's care is vast. If successful, gene editing could lead to **personalized treatments** that address the genetic risk factors of individual patients, offering a more tailored approach to preventing or slowing the disease.

Stem Cell Therapy: Regenerating Brain Cells

Stem cell therapy is another emerging area of research that offers the potential to regenerate damaged brain cells in people with Alzheimer's. Stem cells are unique in that they can differentiate into various types of cells, including neurons. By harnessing the power of stem cells, researchers hope to replace or repair the neurons that are lost or damaged in Alzheimer's disease, ultimately restoring cognitive function.

How Stem Cell Therapy Works

Pluripotent stem cells, which can develop into any type of cell in the body, can be transformed into **neuronal cells** in the lab. These newly created neurons can then be transplanted into the brains of Alzheimer's patients with the goal of replacing the neurons that have been lost to the disease.

Mesenchymal stem cells (MSCs). Beyond neural regeneration, mesenchymal stem cells (MSCs) harvested from bone marrow act as cellular pharmacies, releasing powerful neurotrophic factors that nourish struggling neurons and potentially halt their death - addressing Alzheimer's fundamental problem of neural loss rather than just its symptoms.

Progress in Stem Cell Research for Alzheimer's

Early clinical trials have shown that stem cell therapy may have a positive impact on brain function and cognitive abilities in Alzheimer's patients. In animal models, stem cell transplants have been shown to reduce amyloid plaques, improve memory, and promote the regeneration of neural connections.

One promising approach involves induced pluripotent stem cells (iPSCs), which are derived from adult cells (such as skin cells) and reprogrammed to behave like embryonic stem cells. iPSCs can be turned into neurons and used to study Alzheimer's disease in a laboratory setting, helping researchers understand how the disease progresses and test new treatments. Additionally, iPSCs have the potential to be used for personalized cell therapies, where a patient's own cells are reprogrammed to create new neurons and then transplanted into the brain.

Challenges and Potential of Stem Cell Therapy

Successful stem cell therapy requires more than simply depositing new cells into damaged brain regions - these transplanted neurons must navigate the bewildering complexity of forming precisely the right connections with existing neural networks, similar to adding new musicians to an orchestra mid-symphony without disrupting the performance. The brain is a highly complex and delicate organ, and simply introducing new neurons is not enough - they must be able to communicate effectively with other cells to restore cognitive function.

Another challenge is the long-term safety of stem cell therapies. Researchers are still exploring how these therapies behave over time, including the risk of abnormal cell growth or rejection by the patient's immune system. Additionally, stem cell treatments are still in the experimental stages, and much more research is needed to determine their efficacy and safety for Alzheimer's patients.

Despite these hurdles, stem cell therapy holds tremendous potential as a regenerative treatment for Alzheimer's. By replacing lost neurons and repairing damaged brain tissue, stem cell therapy could help restore cognitive function and slow the progression of the disease.

Combining Gene Editing and Stem Cell Therapies with Existing Treatments

Both gene editing and stem cell therapies are still in the early stages of development, but they could eventually be combined with existing Alzheimer's treatments, such as immunotherapy and neuroprotective drugs, to create a multi-faceted approach to Alzheimer's care. For example:

Immunotherapy treatments, which use the body's immune system to target and remove amyloid plaques or tau tangles, could be used in conjunction with gene editing to reduce the production of these proteins at the genetic level.

Neuroprotective drugs that aim to protect neurons from damage could complement stem cell therapies by creating a more supportive environment for newly transplanted cells, ensuring their survival and integration into the brain.

Combining these emerging therapies with current

treatments could result in a more comprehensive approach to Alzheimer's care, targeting multiple aspects of the disease at once and potentially offering greater benefits to patients.

The Future of Emerging Therapies in Alzheimer's Care

While gene editing and stem cell therapies hold great promise, they are still in the experimental phase, and more research is needed to determine their long-term effectiveness and safety. However, the potential for these therapies to modify the course of Alzheimer's disease is significant.

From Laboratory Promise to Clinical Reality: Key Milestones to Watch

Ongoing clinical trials: Current clinical trials are testing the safety and efficacy of both gene editing and stem cell therapies in humans. As more data becomes available, researchers will gain a clearer understanding of how these therapies can be used in Alzheimer's care and whether they can provide lasting cognitive benefits.

Personalized medicine: In the future, gene editing and stem cell therapies could become key components of personalized Alzheimer's care, where treatments are tailored to an individual's genetic makeup and specific disease pathology. This personalized approach could lead to more effective interventions that target the root causes of Alzheimer's in each patient.

Emerging therapies such as gene editing and stem cell treatments represent the next frontier in Alzheimer's research, offering the potential to not only slow the progression of the disease but also to address its root causes at the genetic and cellular levels. While these therapies are still in the early stages of development, they hold tremendous promise for transforming the future of Alzheimer's care. As research continues, these groundbreaking therapies could one day provide patients and families with new hope for effective treatments and even the possibility of reversing the damage caused by Alzheimer's disease.

What Can Be Done to Ensure Equitable Access to Alzheimer's Treatments Across Diverse Communities?

Access to advanced Alzheimer's treatments and technologies often varies based on a patient's geographic location, socioeconomic status, race, ethnicity, and other factors. These disparities result in unequal opportunities for diagnosis, treatment, and participation in clinical trials, leaving certain communities underserved and at a higher risk for poor health outcomes. As Alzheimer's treatments continue to evolve, it is crucial to ensure that all patients - regardless of background - have equitable access to the best possible care. Governments, healthcare systems, and advocacy groups must work together to address systemic barriers and create a more inclusive healthcare landscape for Alzheimer's patients.

1. Addressing Geographic Disparities in Access to Care

One of the most significant barriers to equitable Alzheimer's care is geographic location. In rural and underserved areas, access to specialized Alzheimer's care - such as memory clinics, neurologists, or clinical trials - is often limited. Patients in these areas may have to travel long distances to receive a diagnosis or access advanced treatments, creating a substantial burden for families already dealing with the challenges of caregiving.

Solutions to Reduce Geographic Disparities

- **Telemedicine and Remote Care**: The expansion of telemedicine can bridge the gap between rural patients and Alzheimer's specialists. By using virtual consultations and remote monitoring technologies, patients can receive expert care without needing to travel to distant healthcare facilities. Telemedicine also allows for regular follow-ups and personalized care plans, ensuring that patients in underserved areas receive ongoing support.

- **Mobile Health Clinics**: Mobile health clinics that travel to rural and underserved communities can provide on-the-ground Alzheimer's screenings, diagnoses, and early interventions. These clinics can offer cognitive assessments, educational resources, and referrals to specialized care, making it easier for patients to access services that may otherwise be out of reach.

- **Partnerships with Local Healthcare Providers**: By training local healthcare providers - including general practitioners, nurses, and community health workers - in Alzheimer's care, healthcare systems can expand access to diagnosis and treatment. Establishing partnerships between large medical centers and local providers allows for greater collaboration and increases the reach of specialized services

2. Improving Access for Low-Income Patients

Socioeconomic status plays a significant role in determining access to Alzheimer's treatments. Low-income patients often face financial barriers that prevent them from receiving timely diagnoses, affording treatments, or participating in clinical trials. Without adequate insurance coverage or the means to pay out-of-pocket costs, many families struggle to access the best care.

Solutions to Improve Access for Low-Income Patients:

- **Expanding Insurance Coverage**: Governments can work to ensure that Medicare, Medicaid, and private insurance plans provide comprehensive coverage for Alzheimer's care, including early screenings, cognitive testing, and long-term treatment options. Policies that reduce copays, cover new medications, and provide financial support for caregivers can make advanced treatments more accessible to low-income patients.

- **Subsidized Treatment Programs**: Pharmaceutical companies, in partnership with governments and nonprofit organizations, can create subsidized treatment **programs** that provide medications and therapies at reduced or no cost for low-income patients. These programs can be critical for ensuring that the latest Alzheimer's treatments are not limited to those who can afford them.

- **Financial Assistance for Clinical Trials**: Participation in clinical trials is often financially out of reach for low-income patients due to travel costs, missed workdays, and caregiving responsibilities. Offering financial assistance for trial **participation**, including travel stipends, caregiver support, and compensation for time, can help remove these barriers and increase the diversity of clinical trial participants.

3. Addressing Racial and Ethnic Disparities in Alzheimer's Care

Research shows that certain racial and ethnic groups - such as African Americans and Hispanic/Latino communities - are disproportionately affected by Alzheimer's and other forms of dementia. African Americans, for instance, are about twice as likely as white Americans to develop Alzheimer's, while Hispanics/Latinos are about 1.5 times more likely. Despite this elevated risk, these groups are often underdiagnosed and underrepresented in clinical trials, leading to significant disparities in access to care and treatment.

Solutions to Address Racial and Ethnic Disparities

Addressing racial and ethnic disparities in healthcare,

particularly in the diagnosis and treatment of Alzheimer's, is essential for ensuring equitable access to quality care. Research has shown that minority populations, including Black, Hispanic, and Indigenous communities, are disproportionately affected by Alzheimer's and related dementias, yet they often face barriers to early diagnosis, treatment, and support services. These disparities stem from a range of factors, including socioeconomic challenges, cultural stigma, healthcare access, and historical mistrust of medical institutions. To bridge this gap, targeted solutions must be implemented, such as increasing diversity in clinical trials, expanding community outreach and education, improving cultural competency in healthcare, and addressing social determinants of health. By tackling these challenges head-on, we can move toward a more inclusive healthcare system that ensures every individual, regardless of race or ethnicity, receives the care and support they deserve

- **Culturally Competent Care**: Healthcare systems must prioritize culturally competent care that addresses the unique needs and concerns of diverse populations. This includes training healthcare providers to recognize the specific ways that Alzheimer's may manifest in different racial and ethnic groups and ensuring that language barriers do not prevent patients from accessing care. Culturally tailored education and outreach programs can also help raise awareness about Alzheimer's within these communities, promoting early detection and intervention.
- **Increasing Diversity in Clinical Trials**: Ensuring that clinical trials are inclusive of diverse racial and ethnic populations is essential for developing treatments that are effective for all patients. Researchers and trial sponsors must actively recruit participants from underrepresented groups and work with

community leaders to build trust and promote trial participation. Offering language support, culturally relevant materials, and transportation assistance can help increase participation from historically underserved communities.

- **Community-Based Interventions**: Partnering with community organizations and faith-based groups can help healthcare systems reach communities that may be skeptical of mainstream healthcare institutions due to past discrimination or lack of trust. These partnerships can provide valuable education on Alzheimer's prevention, diagnosis, and treatment, as well as connect patients with local resources and support networks.

4. Reducing the Cost of New Alzheimer's Treatments

New Alzheimer's treatments, particularly advanced therapies such as monoclonal antibodies or emerging technologies like gene editing and stem cell treatments, are often expensive and out of reach for many patients. As these therapies become available, it is critical to ensure that they are affordable and accessible to all who need them.

Solutions to Reduce Treatment Costs

The high cost of Alzheimer's treatment places a significant financial burden on patients, families, and healthcare systems, making it crucial to explore solutions that reduce expenses while ensuring quality care. From the cost of medications and long-term care to specialized therapies and caregiver support, managing Alzheimer's can quickly become overwhelming. Addressing these financial challenges requires a multi-pronged approach, including expanding insurance coverage, increasing access to government assistance programs like Medicare and Medicaid, promoting the development of more affordable generic medications, and investing in community-based care options. Additionally, advancements in AI and telemedicine have the potential to lower diagnostic and treatment costs by improving early detection and enabling remote patient monitoring. By implementing these solutions, we can work toward making Alzheimer's care more accessible and affordable, easing the financial strain on families while improving patient outcomes.

- **Government Negotiation of Drug Prices**: Allowing governments to negotiate the **prices** of new Alzheimer's medications can help make treatments more affordable for patients. Countries with single-payer healthcare systems often have more leverage in setting prices, but even in countries like the U.S., recent legislation has opened the door for Medicare to negotiate prices on high-cost drugs, which could include Alzheimer's treatments.

- **Value-Based Pricing Models**: Implementing value-based pricing - where the price of a drug is tied to its clinical effectiveness - can help ensure that patients are paying a fair price for treatments. This model incentivizes pharmaceutical companies to develop highly effective treatments while ensuring that patients benefit from lower costs if the treatment is not as effective as anticipated.

- **Generic and Biosimilar Medications**: As patents for Alzheimer's drugs expire, encouraging the development of generic or biosimilar versions of these medications can significantly reduce costs. Governments can fast-track the approval of these alternatives to increase market competition and make advanced treatments more affordable.

5. Increasing Awareness and Education in Underserved Communities

Many underserved communities are unaware of the symptoms of Alzheimer's or the importance of early diagnosis, leading to delayed treatment and worse outcomes. Raising awareness about Alzheimer's within these communities is key to ensuring equitable access to care.

Solutions to Increase Awareness

- **Public Health Campaigns**: Governments and nonprofit organizations can create targeted public health campaigns to raise awareness about Alzheimer's in underserved communities. These campaigns should be delivered in multiple languages and through culturally relevant channels, such as community centers, churches, and local media outlets.

- **Education for Primary Care Providers**: Education for Primary Care Providers: Primary care providers serve as critical frontline detectors of cognitive decline, yet many lack specialized training in recognizing how Alzheimer's manifests differently across cultural and ethnic groups. Implementing mandatory continuing education in culturally sensitive cognitive assessment can dramatically improve early detection rates in underserved communities where specialized neurological care is often inaccessible.

- **Support for Caregivers in Underserved Communities**: Many underserved families face significant challenges in caring for loved ones with Alzheimer's, including a lack of financial resources, time, and access to support services. Offering free or low-cost caregiving support, such as respite care, counseling, and caregiver training, can help alleviate the burden on these families and ensure that patients receive the care they need.

6. Advocating for Policy Changes to Promote

Equitable Access

Policy changes at the national and local levels are critical to ensuring that all patients, regardless of background, have access to the latest Alzheimer's treatments and technologies.

Key Policy Actions

- **Increasing Funding for Alzheimer's Research**: Governments should prioritize funding for Alzheimer's research, with a focus on developing treatments that are effective for diverse populations. Additionally, funding should be directed toward improving access to care in rural and underserved communities.

- **Expanding Alzheimer's Centers of Excellence**: Governments can create more Alzheimer's Centers of Excellence in underserved areas, where patients can access specialized care, participate in clinical trials, and receive support services. These centers can also serve as hubs for community outreach and education.

- **Creating National Alzheimer's Care Plans**: National Alzheimer's care plans that include provisions for equitable access can help ensure that healthcare systems prioritize inclusivity. These plans can set goals for reducing disparities in diagnosis, treatment, and clinical trial participation while creating accountability mechanisms to track progress.

Ensuring equitable access to Alzheimer's treatments across diverse communities is critical for addressing the growing burden of the disease. By expanding access to care through telemedicine, improving insurance coverage, addressing racial and ethnic disparities, and reducing the cost of treatments, healthcare systems and governments can work together to create a more inclusive healthcare landscape. Raising awareness and advocating for policy changes will further help eliminate barriers and ensure that all patients - regardless of geography, income, or background - have access to the best possible Alzheimer's care and emerging treatments.

What Lessons Can Be Learned from Past Research Failures to Improve Future Alzheimer's Studies?

. Despite pouring decades of intensive research and billions of dollars into finding a cure, Alzheimer's continues to outmaneuver our best scientific minds. The journey to find effective treatments has been fraught with setbacks, particularly in clinical trials that have failed to meet their endpoints. However, these past failures offer valuable insights that can inform future research efforts, guiding scientists toward more promising strategies. By learning from the mistakes and challenges of past studies, researchers can refine their approaches, increase the likelihood of breakthroughs, and ultimately advance the fight against Alzheimer's.

1. Revisiting the Amyloid Hypothesis: A Need for Broader Focus

Research has been dominated by a singular focus on the amyloid hypothesis - the theory that protein plaques accumulating in the brain drive the disease - which has led us down an increasingly narrow path with diminishing returns. This theory has led to the development of numerous drugs aimed at reducing amyloid plaques. Unfortunately, most of these drugs have failed to show meaningful clinical benefits in large-scale trials.

Lessons Learned

Amyloid may not be the sole cause: While amyloid plaques are a hallmark of Alzheimer's, the failure of amyloid-targeting drugs suggests that other factors may also play critical roles in the disease. Tau tangles, inflammation, and vascular changes in the brain are increasingly recognized as contributing factors. Future research should take a multifactorial approach by targeting not only amyloid but also tau proteins, neuroinflammation, and other pathological processes that may drive Alzheimer's.

Earlier intervention may be key: Many amyloid-targeting drugs were tested in patients who already had moderate to severe Alzheimer's, which may have been too late to make a significant impact. Recent studies suggest that amyloid plaques begin accumulating in the brain years before symptoms appear. Future trials should focus on early-stage or preclinical patients, who may benefit more from interventions that prevent or slow the onset of cognitive decline before significant damage has occurred.

2. Understanding the Complexity of Alzheimer's Pathology

Alzheimer's is a highly complex disease with multiple overlapping pathways contributing to cognitive decline. Research that focuses on a single target or mechanism has often failed to address the full scope of the disease.

Multimodal therapies may be more effective: The failures of single-target drugs suggest that a combination of therapies targeting multiple aspects of Alzheimer's pathology could yield better results. For example, drugs that reduce amyloid plaques could be combined with therapies that target tau tangles or reduce neuroinflammation. By **combining treatments** that address different pathways, researchers may be able to slow or halt the progression of the disease more effectively.

Genetic and environmental diversity matters: Alzheimer's affects individuals differently based on their genetic makeup, lifestyle, and environmental factors. Previous trials often overlooked this diversity, leading to treatments that may not work for all patients. Going forward, researchers should consider **personalized medicine approaches**, tailoring treatments to individual patients based on genetic risk factors like the APOE ε4 allele or other biomarkers.

3. The Importance of Early Detection and Biomarkers

One of the biggest challenges in Alzheimer's research has been the difficulty of diagnosing the disease in its earliest stages, when interventions may be most effective. Many clinical trials have failed because they included patients whose disease was too advanced for treatments to work.

Improved diagnostic tools: Future research should focus on developing better biomarkers for early detection of Alzheimer's. This could include more sensitive blood tests, cerebrospinal fluid tests, or advanced imaging techniques that can detect amyloid or tau buildup long before symptoms appear. Early diagnosis would allow for earlier intervention, which is critical for slowing disease progression.

Focus on preclinical and early-stage patients: Trials should increasingly recruit individuals in the preclinical or early-stage phase of Alzheimer's, when interventions are more likely to be effective. This shift in focus could lead to better outcomes in clinical trials and increase the likelihood of finding treatments that can delay or prevent the onset of symptoms.

4. Rethinking Clinical Trial Design

Many Alzheimer's clinical trials have failed to demonstrate significant effects, partly due to flaws in trial design. The traditional clinical trial model - designed for diseases with straightforward mechanisms and rapid progression - fundamentally mismatches Alzheimer's complex, decades-long development, demanding entirely new approaches to how we test potential treatments.

Adaptive trial designs: Traditional randomized controlled trials can be rigid and slow, making it difficult to test multiple treatments simultaneously. Adaptive trial designs, such as those used in the European Prevention of Alzheimer's Dementia (EPAD) initiative, allow researchers to test multiple interventions at once and adjust protocols in response to interim results. These flexible designs could reduce trial durations and costs while increasing the chances of identifying effective treatments.

Longer trial durations: Alzheimer's disease progresses slowly, and the effects of treatments may take years to become apparent. Some past trials may have been too short to detect meaningful differences between treated and placebo groups. Future trials should consider longer follow-up periods to capture the full impact of therapies over time.

Enriching trial populations: Recruiting patients who are at higher risk of Alzheimer's, based on biomarkers or genetic factors, can increase the likelihood of detecting treatment effects. This enrichment strategy allows researchers to focus on individuals who are more likely to benefit from the intervention, making trials more efficient and increasing the chances of success.

5. Fostering Collaboration and Data Sharing

Alzheimer's research has often been fragmented, with different institutions and pharmaceutical companies conducting trials independently. This lack of collaboration has led to duplication of efforts, wasted resources, and missed opportunities to learn from both successes and failures.

Collaborative research networks: Future Alzheimer's research can benefit from greater collaboration between academic institutions, pharmaceutical companies, and government agencies. By working together and sharing data, researchers can accelerate the pace of discovery and avoid redundant trials. Initiatives like the Global Alzheimer's Association Interactive Network (GAAIN), which provides an open platform for sharing Alzheimer's research data, are a step in the right direction.

Open access to trial data: Many past Alzheimer's trials have failed, but the data collected from those failures can still provide valuable insights. Researchers should make clinical trial data - including from failed trials - more accessible to the scientific community. Sharing data allows researchers to analyze what went wrong, identify potential signals that were missed, and design better future studies.

6. Engaging Diverse Patient Populations

One of the major limitations of past Alzheimer's research has been the underrepresentation of diverse populations in clinical trials. Many trials have predominantly enrolled white, Western participants, which limits the generalizability of the findings to other racial and ethnic groups.

Diversity in clinical trials: To ensure that new treatments are effective for all patients, future trials must include more diverse populations, including people of different racial, ethnic, and socioeconomic backgrounds. This diversity is essential for understanding how Alzheimer's affects different groups and for developing treatments that are broadly effective.

Community outreach and education: Researchers should engage with underserved communities to raise awareness about Alzheimer's research and encourage participation in clinical trials. This could involve partnering with local healthcare providers, community leaders, and advocacy groups to build trust and educate potential participants about the benefits of joining clinical studies.

7. Addressing the Need for a Holistic Approach

Alzheimer's disease is not just a neurological condition - it is influenced by factors such as cardiovascular health, diet, exercise, and social engagement. Past research has often focused too narrowly on single biological targets, without considering the broader context of overall health.

Holistic approaches: Future research should explore multidisciplinary approaches to Alzheimer's prevention and treatment. For example, combining lifestyle interventions - such as improved diet, regular exercise, and cognitive training - with pharmacological treatments could offer a more comprehensive strategy for managing the disease. Ongoing studies, such as the FINGER study in Finland, are already exploring the benefits of combined lifestyle and medical interventions, and these efforts should be expanded.

A Message of Hope

Our collective scientific failures in Alzheimer's research, properly understood, aren't endpoints but essential steppingstones - each unsuccessful trial narrows the field of possibilities and illuminates paths not yet taken, gradually leading us toward approaches that embrace the disease's true complexity. By adopting a more multifaceted approach - targeting not only amyloid but also tau, inflammation, and other pathways - researchers can develop more effective treatments. Improved diagnostic tools, early intervention, diverse clinical trials, and collaborative research networks will be critical for accelerating breakthroughs. With these insights, the Alzheimer's research community is better equipped to overcome the challenges of the past and bring us closer to finding a cure for this devastating disease

Alzheimer's is more than a disease; it is a profound journey that reshapes the lives of those it touches. From the initial signs of forgetfulness to the poignant fragility of lucid moments, the path is filled with challenges that test our resilience, patience, and love. Yet, it is also a journey that inspires innovation, fosters deep connections, and calls forth the best of human compassion.

Throughout this book, we've explored the complex layers of Alzheimer's: its neurological roots, its emotional and practical toll, the stigma it carries, and the promising horizons of medical and technological advancements. At its core, this story is about people - those living with Alzheimer's, their caregivers, and the global community united in the fight to understand and overcome it.

As science marches forward with breakthroughs in early diagnosis, personalized medicine, and emerging therapies, there is real hope on the horizon. Each discovery brings us closer to a world where Alzheimer's is no longer a devastating diagnosis but a manageable condition - or one that can be prevented entirely. The integration of technology, though fraught with ethical challenges, holds immense potential to transform care, making it safer, more effective, and more compassionate.

But hope doesn't rest solely in the hands of researchers and medical professionals. It rests with each of us. By challenging stigma, advocating for equity, and supporting caregivers, we can create a culture of understanding and inclusion. Families navigating this journey need more than treatment; they need a community that walks alongside them, offering empathy, resources, and strength.

A Future of Possibility

The road ahead is not without obstacles, but it is illuminated by the unwavering dedication of those who refuse to give up - scientists, caregivers, advocates, and individuals like you who seek to make a difference. Together, we can envision a future where memories lost to Alzheimer's are replaced by stories of triumph, innovation, and connection.

As you close this book, may you carry with you a sense of purpose: to honor the lives of those affected by Alzheimer's, to support the caregivers who tirelessly give of themselves, and to contribute, in whatever way you can, to a brighter, more compassionate future

"Alzheimer's may steal memories, but it cannot erase the enduring power of love, humanity, and hope."

ACKNOWLEDGMENTS

Writing this book has been an emotional journey - one filled with deep reflection, heartache, and hope. I could not have completed it without the love, support, and encouragement of so many people who have walked beside me through this experience.

First and foremost, I want to express my deepest gratitude to my husband, whose unwavering love and understanding provided me with the strength to put these words on paper. Your support has been my anchor during the most challenging moments.

To my family, especially my dear Claire, whose life and struggles with Alzheimer's inspired this book - this is for you. Your journey has taught me about resilience, patience, and the profound depth of love that endures even when memories fade.

To the caregivers and medical professionals who dedicate their lives to supporting those with Alzheimer's - you are true heroes. Your compassion and commitment bring comfort to so many families navigating the heartbreak of this disease.

To my friends and fellow writers, thank you for listening, offering feedback, and reminding me why sharing this story is so important. Your encouragement kept me motivated when the weight of the topic felt overwhelming.

And to my readers - those who have experienced the impact of Alzheimer's firsthand or who seek to understand it better - thank you for allowing me to share this journey with you. I hope these pages bring you comfort, insight, and a sense of solidarity.

Finally, I am grateful for the resilience of the human spirit, for the moments of clarity that remind us that love transcends memory, and for the hope that continues to shine even in the darkest times.

With heartfelt appreciation,
Maria L. Ellis, BBA, MBA

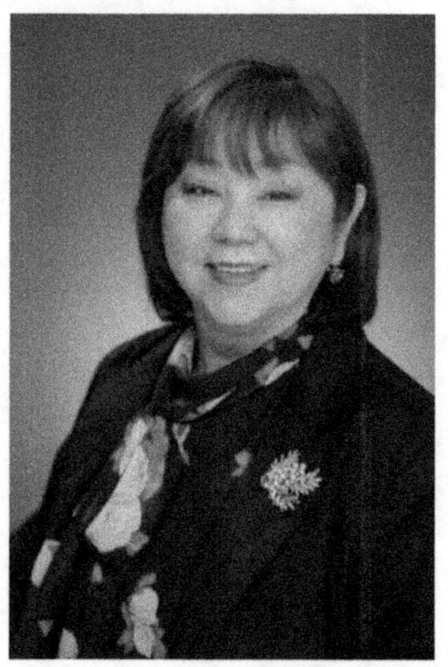

Maria L. Ellis, MBA, is a graduate of the Harvard Business School Owner-President Management Program and earned her bachelor's degree in business administration as well as her MBA from the University of Massachusetts in Amherst. As a former international banker, investment advisor, and financial planner, Maria has specialized in converting clients' financial objectives into successful action plans. Maria has both the know-how and the market contacts, having worked at Bank of America, Citibank, the MONY Group, Northwestern Mutual, Citi Habitats and Keller Williams.

Maria is a Chopra Certified Health Instructor, and she is the bestselling author of the Journey to Wellness, Freedom, and Legacy series, which includes *Achieve Financial Freedom: The Road Map to Financial Success*; *Family Business Legacy Plan: The Ultimate Guide to Creating a Legacy for Your Family without Paying too Much in Taxes*; *Redefining Entrepreneurial Success: A Guide to a Healthy and Holistic Lifestyle*; *Longevity: Reinvent Yourself at Any Age*; *Life on Earth: Poetic Perspectives*; *Golf: A Course in Business: A Few Lessons Golf Can Teach Us about Management and Entrepreneurship*; and *From Operator to Entrepreneur: Unlocking the Power of Visionary Leadership*.

Maria's background includes board leadership positions at the College of Mount Saint Vincent, the American Association of University Women, and the Virginia Gildersleeve International Fund. Maria is also a pro-bono consultant at the Harvard Business School Club of New York City Community Partners and applies her business skills to a variety of topics, including strategic planning, marketing, finance, governance, and organizational development. Maria is an active member of the Harvard Club and the Genuis Network.

THANK YOU!

Dear Reader,

Thank you for picking up *Stolen Memories: A Journey Through Alzheimer's*. Writing this book has been a deeply personal and emotional experience, and I am honored to share it with you.

Alzheimer's is a cruel disease - one that steals moments, relationships, and identities. Yet, through the pain and loss, it also reveals the power of love, patience, and resilience. Whether you are reading this as a caregiver, a family member, or simply someone seeking to understand, please know that you are not alone.

I want to express my deepest gratitude to those who dedicate their lives to caring for individuals with Alzheimer's. Your kindness and commitment bring comfort and dignity to so many. To the families navigating this journey, I see you. I know the heartbreak, the exhaustion, and the small, bittersweet joys found in fleeting moments of recognition.

This book is my tribute to those we have lost and to those still fighting - both the patients and their loved ones. My hope is that these words bring you comfort, validation, and perhaps even a sense of peace as you walk this path.

Thank you for allowing me to share this journey with you. I encourage you to share your own stories, to continue raising awareness, and most importantly, to hold onto love, even when memories fade.

With gratitude,
Maria L. Ellis, BBA, MBA.

www.ingramcontent.com/pod-product-compliance
Lightning Source LLC
Chambersburg PA
CBHW051413050726
47595CB00010B/4042